PROMOTING HEALTH

Report of the Task Force
on
Consumer Health Education

Anne R. Somers, Chairman

Sponsored by:
The John E. Fogarty International Center
for Advanced Studies in the Health Sciences
National Institutes of Health
and
The American College of Preventive Medicine

PROMOTING HEALTH

Consumer Education and National Policy

Anne R. Somers, Editor

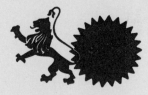

AN ASPEN PUBLICATION

Library of Congress Catalog Card Number: 76-21444
ISBN: 0-912862-25-4

Printed in the United States of America.

345

To the Memory of
Fred R. McCrumb, Jr., M.D.
1925–1976

Table Of Contents

Task Force IV
Consumer Health Education

Chairman
Anne R. Somers
Associate Professor
of Community Medicine
College of Medicine and Dentistry of New Jersey
Rutgers Medical School
Piscataway, New Jersey 08854

Barbara Echols Anlyan
Director
Office of Grants, Contracts &
   Special Projects
Duke University Medical School
Durham, North Carolina 27705

Avon Arnold
Executive Director
Planned Parenthood Association of
   Mercer County
211 Academy Street
Trenton, New Jersey 08608

Mary Ashley
Department of Community
   Medicine
Charles R. Drew Postgraduate
   Medical School
1635 E. 103d Street
Los Angeles, California 90002

Frederick Bass, M.D.
Vancouver Health Department
1060 W. 8th Avenue
Vancouver, B.C., Canada

Richard Bates, M.D.
Director

Alcoholism Clinic
Sparrow Hospital
Lansing, Michigan 48912

Robert Cunningham, Jr.
Chairman
Editorial Board
Modern Healthcare
Chicago, Illinois 60606

Thomas D. Dublin, M.D.
Special Assistant to the Director
Bureau of Health Resources
   Development
Building 31, Room 3C11
National Institutes of Health
Bethesda, Maryland 20014

John Knowles, M.D.
President
The Rockefeller Foundation
111 West 50th Street
New York, New York 10021

Nathan Maccoby, Ph.D.
Chairman, Institute of
   Communication Research
Co-Director, Stanford Heart
   Disease Prevention Program

Stanford University Medical
  Center
Stanford, California 94305

Walter McNerney
President
Blue Cross Association
840 N. Lake Shore Drive
Chicago, Illinois 60611

Carter L. Marshall, M.D.
Associate Dean
Mt. Sinai School of Medicine
The City University of New York
Fifth Avenue and 100th Street
New York, New York 10029

Dorothy Novella, R.N., Ph.D.
Dean
Erie Institute of Nursing
Villa Maria College
2551 W. Lake Road
Erie, Pennsylvania 16505

Richard Podell, M.D.
Associate Director of Family
  Practice Education
Overlook Hospital
Summit, New Jersey 07901

Irving S. Shapiro, Ph.D.

Director
Health Education Program
School of Public Health
Columbia University
600 W. 168th Street
New York, New York 10032

Scott K. Simonds, Dr. P.H.
Director of Health Education
  Programs
University of Michigan School of
  Public Health
Ann Arbor, Michigan 48104

Harvey T. Stephens*
Chairman
World Food Systems, Inc.
1707 L Street, N.W.
Washington, D.C. 20036

Earl Ubell, Ph.D.
News Director
WNBC TV—New York
300 Rockefeller Center
New York, New York 10020

Paul Norman Ylvisaker, Ph.D.
Dean
Graduate School of Education
Harvard University
Cambridge, Massachusettes 02138

EX OFFICIO

Fred R. McCrumb, Jr., M.D.**
Special Assistant to the Director
Fogarty International Center
National Institutes of Health
Bethesda, Maryland 20014

Toby P. Levin
Special Assistant
Conference and Seminar Program
Fogarty International Center
National Institutes of Health
Bethesda, Maryland 20014

* Deceased August 1975
**Deceased January 1976

Consumer Health Education
Definition

In view of the frequent inconsistency in use of the terms "health education" and "consumer health education," the Task Force felt it essential to
develop an agreed definition. The following is from Part Three of the Report.
The term "consumer health education" subsumes a set of six activities
that —

1. inform people about health, illness, disability, and ways in which they
can improve and protect their own health, including more efficient use of
the delivery system;
2. motivate people to want to change to more healthful practices;
3. help them to learn the necessary skills to adopt and maintain healthful
practices and life styles;
4. foster teaching and communication skills in all those engaged in educating consumers about health;
5. advocate changes in the environment that will facilitate healthful conditions and healthful behavior; and
6. add to knowledge through research and evaluation concerning the
most effective ways of achieving these objectives.

In brief, consumer health education (CHE) is a process that informs, mo-
tivates, and helps people to adopt and maintain healthy practices and life
styles, advocates the environmental changes needed to facilitate this goal,
and conducts professional training and research to the same end.

Acknowledgments

The Task Force is indebted to a number of individuals at NIH Fogarty International Center who helped with our deliberations and the preparation of this report, especially Dr. Fred McCrumb, Special Assistant to the Director until his death in January 1976; Toby P. Levin, Conference Management Assistant; and Michiko Cooper, Conference Coordinator.

At the American College of Preventive Medicine, three successive presidents—Dr. Kurt W. Deuschle, Dr. Mary McLaughlin, and Dr. Irving Tabershaw—and Ward Bentley, Executive Director, provided continuous support and encouragement.

Joanne Hilferty and John Weingart, students at Princeton University's Woodrow Wilson School of Public and International Affairs, assisted in preparation of the first draft of this report. Laura Stabler and, later, Lois Walker helped the chairman as administrative assistants. Thelma Shays and Linda Mento did the typing.

To all these individuals we wish to express our appreciation for their interest and their efforts, which went far beyond their formal duties.

Introduction

On June 23, 1976, President Ford signed into law P.L. 94–317. Title I—the National Consumer Health Information and Health Promotion Act of 1976—provides for a national program of "health information, health promotion, preventive health services, and education in the appropriate use of health care."

The Secretary of Health, Education, and Welfare is instructed to formulate national goals with respect to these four broad areas and a strategy to achieve such goals and to support programs to carry out the strategy. (For the full text of Title I, see Appendix W.)

Following are among the specific duties assigned to the Secretary:

- "to incorporate appropriate health education components into our society, especially into all aspects of education and health care";
- "to increase the application and use of health knowledge, skills, and practices by the general population in its patterns of daily living";
- "to establish systematic processes for the exploration, development, demonstration, and evaluation of innovative health promotion concepts";
- to undertake and support, by grant or contract, research and demonstration programs in the four areas—health information, health promotion, preventive health services, and education in the appropriate use of health care—including "environmental, occupational, social, and behavioral factors which affect and determine health"; "methods of disseminating information concerning personal health behavior, preventive health services and the appropriate use of health care and of affecting behavior so that such information is applied to maintain and improve health"; methods by which the cost and effectiveness of such activities can be measured, evaluated, standardized, and paid for; and "methods for assessing the cost

and effectiveness of specific medical services and procedures . . . including screening and diagnostic procedures";

● to undertake and support (and encourage others to support) new and innovative programs in the four areas, including community programs based in hospitals, ambulatory and home care settings, schools, day care programs, voluntary health agencies, medical societies, and other private nonprofit health organizations;

● to develop health information and health promotion materials and teaching programs for both professionals and consumers;

● to support demonstration and evaluation programs for individual and group self-care programs to help the participant maximize his potential for dealing with health problems, including obesity, hypertension, and diabetes;

● to make grants to states and other nonprofit organizations for support of demonstration and evaluation programs "which provide information respecting the costs and quality of health care or information respecting health insurance policies and prepaid plans";

● to support the publication of informational material pertaining to the four areas, including "child care, family life and human development, disease prevention (particularly prevention of pulmonary disease, cardiovascular disease, and cancer), physical fitness, dental health, environmental health, nutrition, safety and accident prevention, drug abuse and alcoholism, mental health, management of chronic diseases (including diabetes and arthritis), and venereal diseases";

● to secure "the cooperation of the communications media . . . in activities designed to promote and encourage the use of health maintaining information and behavior";

● to study health information and promotion in advertising and recommend to federal agencies and others appropriate action with respect to such advertising;

● to recommend appropriate educational and quality assurance measures for the manpower needed to carry out the above programs;

● to make a periodic survey of the needs, attitudes, and knowledge of United States citizens regarding health care; and

● to conduct a study to determine the extent of health insurance coverage for preventive health services and health education.

THE OFFICE OF HEALTH INFORMATION AND HEALTH PROMOTION

A new Office of Health Information and Health Promotion (OHIHP) is to be established within the Office of the Assistant Secretary for Health. Obviously it is not intended that OHIHP should carry out all the Department functions in the four areas; portions of these responsibilities are already being discharged by the National Institutes of Health, the Center for Disease Control, the National Center for Health Statistics, and other Departmental units. However, the new office is instructed to:

- "coordinate all activities within the Department which relate to health information and health promotion, preventive health services, and education in the appropriate use of health care";
- "coordinate its activities with similar activities of organizations in the private sector"; and
- establish a national health information clearinghouse and analytical center.

The funds authorized for these activities represent a major scaling down from the amounts provided in the original Senate and House legislation. Title I carries a three-year authorization of $31 million: $7 million for fiscal year 1977, $10 million for 1978, and $14 million for 1979.

The significance of the legislation, however, goes far beyond these modest figures. For the first time, the federal government is formally on record as recognizing (1) the crucial roles of individual information, responsibility, and behavior in determining personal and national health status, and (2) the responsibility of government to provide the individual with the necessary information to enable him to advance and protect his own health and to promote social attitudes conducive to motivating people to translate such information into personal practice and life style. It will probably be years before the full implications of this new commitment are fully appreciated, either in government or out. But the first step has been taken. One of the major missing links in United States health policy is beginning to be forged.

ROLE OF THE TASK FORCE

In the course of events that led to this development, the report of the Task Force on Consumer Health Education played a key role. The Task Force was one of eight set up by the Fogarty International Center of the National Institutes of Health and the American College of Preventive Medicine as a strategy for developing a comprehensive program in preventive medicine to be presented to the National Conference on Preventive Medicine held in Washington, D.C., June 1975.

The overall challenge to the Advisory Committee for the conference was presented by Dr. Milo Leavitt, Jr., Director, Fogarty Center, in his opening remarks at the committee's first meeting, August 26, 1974:

> It is obvious even to the casual observer that a huge gap exists between recognition of the virtues of prevention and definition of

ways to accomplish the desired objectives. Therefore, the Department has pledged a full commitment to review of current practice, evaluation of preventive methodology, and the generation of new knowledge. . . .

While the debate will continue as to the precise Federal role in developing and executing a national health plan, most observers recognize the paramount position of the Congress and the Executive in formulating policy guidelines for system reform. There is a unanimous view that a national consensus in preventive medicine is urgently needed for purposes of national health planning.

The charge to the Task Force was as follows:

To explore present day knowledge on the best methods of disseminating information on the value of preventive measures in health care and of effecting behavior so that knowledge is applied to prevent disease, or modify its course or severity.

During discussion at the Advisory Committee's second meeting, September 1974, it was emphasized that the Task Force should take a broad and creative approach to its assignment, that it should not confine itself to the historical concerns of the traditional profession of health education.

In opening our first meeting in Chicago in November 1974, Dr. Robert Stone, Director, NIH, elaborated this point: The Task Force should look beyond the technical issues to broad political forces and constraints. "We are," he said, "in a political ballgame. . . . The name of the process is political. . . . Pure reason is not going to prevail. We've got to use every tool that we can muster in support of what we want to do and what we think is right."

The members of the Task Force were selected with this broad mandate in mind. There were nineteen of us, representing the following diverse backgrounds:

• six physicians, including two practitioners, one foundation president, two medical school faculty, one government administrator;

• four communications experts, including one director of an institute for communications research, one journalist, one news director for a large metropolitan television station, and one physician who also directs a communications program;

• three health educators, including one academic, one practitioner, and one who is both;

• one dean of a school of nursing;

• one dean of a school of education;

• one health insurance executive;

• one medical school administrator and nutritionist;

- one family-planning program director;
- one food industry executive;
- one health economist and health education administrator.

Breadth and diversity were also the major themes of the three meetings between November 1974 and April 1975. The first was held in conjunction with the annual meeting of the Association of American Medical Colleges (AAMC) in Chicago, November 12–14, 1974. In addition to attending the plenary sessions of the AAMC, which were focused entirely on health education, the Task Force met in four separate sessions, and conducted hearings involving twenty representatives of sixteen different organizations engaged in health education or some closely related activity.

At our second meeting, January 1975, we heard from Mr. Larry Fry, Deputy Minister of Health of Canada, Dr. Douglas Niblett, Director General, Community Health Services of Canada, and a representative of the Office of Education, Department of Health, Education, and Welfare.

In addition to these special guests, numerous experts in preventive medicine, health education, and related subjects, from both public and private agencies, attended one or more of our meetings and participated in the discussion. (See Appendix A for the list of witnesses and guests.) The document was circulated, in whole or in part, among numerous interested groups, resulting in a total exposure to several hundred individuals.

In June 1975, it was presented to the National Conference on Preventive Medicine by the chairman and Drs. Bass, Marshall, and Simonds. Invited commentaries were presented by Dr. Jack Elinson, Columbia University School of Public Health, and Dr. Frederick J. Margolis, Wayne State University School of Medicine. A few minor changes were made. In July, at a meeting of the National Advisory Committee, the document was formally approved and its recommendations endorsed on behalf of the National Conference.

ROLE OF CONGRESS AND THE EXECUTIVE

Meanwhile, Congressional initiatives, embodying many of the Task Force recommendations, were already under way. Support was completely bipartisan, coming from Senators Kennedy, Javits, and Schweiker and Congressmen Rogers, Carter, Cohen, and a host of others. Following hearings before the Subcommittee on Health of the Senate Committee on Labor and Public Welfare on May 7–8, 1975, S. 1466 passed the Senate in July. The House approved its version in April 1976. The threat of a Presidential veto led to extensive conferences with the Administration. A compromise measure was accepted by the Senate in May and the House in June, clearing the way for Presidential signature on June 23.

This bare outline does not even suggest the amount of effort that went into the conception, gestation, and birth of this law or the number of individuals who helped in the process. A few must be singled out for special notice: Dr. Arthur Viseltear, Associate Professor of Epidemiology and Public Health, Yale University School of Medicine, and a special legislative assistant to Senator Kennedy and Congressman Carter while serving as a Robert Wood Johnson Fellow in Washington, 1974–75; Dr. Lee Hyde, Staff Assistant, House Subcommittee on Health; Mr. Spencer Johnson, Assistant Director for Health, Social Security, and Welfare, White House Domestic Council; Mr. Donald Carmody, Director, Division of Health Protection, Office of Policy Development and Planning, Office of the Assistant Secretary for Health; and Mr. Gene Haislip, Deputy Assistant Secretary for Legislation (Health), Department of Health, Education, and Welfare.

In November 1975, at the request of the Fogarty Center and the American College of Preventive Medicine (ACPM), the Task Force was reconstituted as an ongoing Expert Panel on Consumer Health Education, responsible to the same two bodies, the Fogarty Center and the ACPM. Dr. Viseltear and Mr. Carmody joined the panel, as well as six additional health professionals engaged in nongovernmental activities and eleven *ex officio* representatives of individual NIH institutes and other HEW units with an interest in health education and health promotion. (For panel membership, see Appendix U.)

The result was a creative and all-too-rare cooperative effort between the Executive, the Congress, and the private sector. All told, passage of P.L. 94–317 came only nineteen months after the Task Force's first meeting in Chicago and twelve months after the National Conference on Preventive Medicine.

Despite passage of P.L. 94–317, the Task Force report is much more than a historic document. In the many compromises that were necessary to secure enactment, several of our recommendations had to be sacrificed or substantially altered. At this point, the Task Force report constitutes an agenda of unfinished business with respect to health education and health promotion.

Perhaps even more important is the problem of implementation. The outcome of the legislation depends very largely on the quality of leadership at OHIHP. Both Senator Kennedy and Congressman Rogers expect the office to be the central locus for policy design, planning, and coordination. With responsibility for harmonizing the health information and health promotion activities of the many autonomous, or semiautonomous, and sometimes warring, bureaus and other units in and out of the federal government, the job calls for the highest level of moral, intellectual, and political, as well as technical, capability. Without such leadership, not only is OHIHP itself likely to be stillborn, but the long and ambitious list of health information and health promotion responsibilities assigned to the department is likely to remain a litany of unfulfilled hopes. In the emergence of the necessary leadership and in the development of a common body of concerns and knowledge, even of a common vocabulary which is still conspicuously missing, the Task Force report can play a useful role.

ORGANIZATION OF THE REPORT

The report is in three parts. Part I emphasizes the relation of health status to life style and the timeliness of the current challenge to consumer health education. Part II summarizes and analyzes current programs, practices, and problems of health education. Part III contains our recommendations.

The appendices are of two types. The majority contain more detailed information on points made in the main body of the report. Several represent studies or proposals advanced by individual Task Force members that we felt should be called to the attention of the Conference, Congress, the Executive. and the general public, but do not necessarily carry the endorsement of the Task Force as a whole.

Total agreement on the wide diversity of topics covered in this report on the part of a Task Force as diverse as ours would patently be impossible and is not necessarily desirable. Both fields, health education and health promotion, are currently in flux—a sign of inherent dynamism—and no one can be sure of having the "single right answer" to any of the many problems involved. Indeed, there probably are no "single right answers."

MAJOR THEMES

With respect to the following major themes, however, the Task Force was in total agreement:

1. Factors of individual behavior and life style play a major role in health, illness, disability, and premature death.

2. Individual behavior and life style are influenced by multiple factors, some of which are internal to the individual and some external—environmental or societal. Health education must address itself to both and hence is intimately related to general policies affecting health.

3. The justification for health education and health promotion depends partly on assumed economies but, even more, on the conviction that good health demands individual knowledge, individual responsibility, and individual participation in making informed choices about one's life. Such individual participation ranges from institutional policymaking to actual health care and behavior changing activities. Addition of the adjective

"consumer" to the older term "health education" in our basic definition and in the title of this report reflects the importance assigned to the consumer role.

4. Health education is not a single discipline but a "field of interest," drawing on knowledge from the biomedical, biostatistical, and behavioral sciences as well as on various administrative, planning, and research skills. Numerous disciplines and would-be disciplines are involved. It is not now possible to say which will emerge as dominant a decade hence.

5. The precise effectiveness of most current health education and health promotion programs and practices is unknown, i.e., the state of the art is still primitive. Substantial empirical research is needed to identify specific and long-term results. However, we learn only by doing and measuring, not by doing nothing. The practice of health education can no more be put off until "all the data are in" than can the practice of medicine. Moreover, there will never be a time when "all the data are in," since the whole context of American society is constantly in flux.

6. Substantial resources should be committed to the advancement of health education and health promotion by both the public and private sectors. Centers of leadership are needed in both sectors.

7. The federal government has a dual responsibility: (a) to promote and assist the development of health education and health promotion; and (b) to take into account the probable effects on health of all major national policies.

8. With respect to health education, as such, the following should be emphasized:

    a. a sustained, rigorous approach to research and development;
    b. a broad-spectrum, decentralized, and regionalized approach to programs and practices;
    c. definition and assistance in meeting manpower needs;
    d. mechanisms for adequate financing; and
    e. incorporation of evaluation into all programs.

It is the hope—both of the Task Force that authored the report and the Expert Panel which is seeking to implement it—that this report will continue to prove a useful guide to policy development in this crucial area, and that our efforts will be helpful to members of Congress, federal and state government officials, the health and education professions, and the American people in general, in meeting the tremendous challenges facing us in the fields of disease prevention, health promotion, and health education.

Princeton, New Jersey   Anne R. Somers
July 26, 1976   Chairman

Part I
Life Style and Health Status:
The Challenge to Health Education

In 1973 hundreds of thousands of Americans died prematurely from causes primarily related to their life style.* Consider the following:

- 757,075 deaths from heart disease
- 115,821 from accidents
- 33,350 from cirrhosis of the liver
- 25,118 from suicide
- 20,465 from homicide[1]

In the same year, death rates for men were 1,073 per 100,000; for women, 814.[2] Life style is an important factor in this difference.

Also in 1973, 13,215 children under age 15 died from accidents or homicide.[3]

It is estimated that $11.5 billion are spent annually in the United States for health care costs associated with cigarette smoking.[4] When both parents smoke, children are twice as likely to get pneumonia or bronchitis in their first year of life as when neither parent smokes.[5]

An estimated nine million Americans are alcoholics or problem drinkers.[6] Drinking among teenagers is now nearly universal, and 36 percent of high school students report getting drunk at least four times a year.[7]

Dr. James McGowan, Director, Alcoholism Services Program, St. Vincent's Hospital in New York City, reports that a 1970 study at the hospital showed that as many as 50 percent of the patients admitted were being treated for illnesses related to alcohol though none had been diagnosed primarily as an alcoholic.[8] Similar or even higher figures are reported for many big city hospitals.

The relationship among death rates, health status, and life style is becoming increasingly clear. Documentation is accumulating at a rapid rate.** Yet individual behavior changes in response to this information

---

*For the purpose of this book, the term "life style" refers only to behavior affecting health.

**For a summary of some preventable health problems and options for action, see "Prevention," excerpt from U.S. Department of Health, Education, and Welfare, *Forward Plan for Health FY 1977-81* in Appendix V.

have been very slow. Smoking, overeating, excessive drinking, and unfastened seat belts are still common facts of American life.

National health policy has been equally slow in responding to changing needs. In fiscal year 1975 Americans paid—in the form of taxes, insurance premiums, and out-of-pocket expenses—an estimated $118.5 billion for health care and related expenses.[9] At the current rate of increase, the figure for FY 1976 will be over $130 billion. Of this staggering total, it is estimated that only 2 to 2.5 percent goes for preventive health measures and .5 percent for health education.[10] Why this anomalous situation?

WHY THE NEGLECT OF CONSUMER
HEALTH EDUCATION?

Throughout recorded history, responsibility for health was placed on the individual. Even primitive tribes prescribed personal practices and tribal tabus related to health. However, as better knowledge of the human body and disease mechanisms were acquired and medical practice became more scientific, society came to place increasing dependence on medical intervention, together with required public health measures. Concomitantly, decreasing emphasis was placed on individual behavior and individual responsibility. Both doctor and patient accepted the authoritarian curative role of the physician as the appropriate avenue to health.

The thirty years since World War II have been particularly difficult for health education. First, the dramatic breakthroughs in polio, chemotherapy, and diagnostic and surgical procedures resulted in an even greater emphasis on professional intervention. "Health" became equated, in the vocabulary of public policy, with "health care."* The pursuit of health was identified almost entirely with professional research, professional care, and more dollars to pay for such care. Care itself was increasingly identified with inpatient care for the acutely ill. Except for a presidentially inspired flurry of interest in physical fitness, the individual's role in his or her own health maintenance has been largely presented in terms of adequate health insurance coverage, access to a physician or hospital, and, in the view of a minority, an annual physical checkup.

Second, as the health care economy grew exponentially during these decades, so did its importance as a source of jobs and livelihood. The health care industry now employs 4.5 million Americans and is one of the two or three largest (depending on the definition). These workers and the professional or-

---

*The phrase "health care" is used throughout this book in the conventional sense although a more accurate term for the activities generally associated therewith would be "disease care."

ganizations and unions that represent them are a powerful constituency for bigger expenditures and for priorities that reflect the interests of the providers rather than the consumers.

Third, the changes in life style that accompanied the unprecedented rise in discretionary income during the sixties and early seventies strongly influenced the health habits and health status of Americans. The rise in income was accompanied by large-scale mass advertising and marketing efforts, appealing to the immediate gratification of pleasure regardless of the consequences for health. Drug advertisers, for example, encourage irresponsibility by assuring Americans that they can "eat, drink, and be merry" to excess as long as they buy "Alka-Seltzer," "Di-Gel," or some other "magic" pill or potion.

Tendencies to carelessness and excess are intensified by conscious and unconscious pressures. Cynicism and apathy, related to a loss of individual and national sense of purpose that resulted in part from Vietnam, Watergate, and the apparently uncontrollable excesses of the American economy, have led many, especially teenagers and young adults, to the pursuit of "La Dolce Vita" without regard for consequences. Deliberate risk taking, always a characteristic of youth, has become a way of life for millions via drugs, "speeding" in both meanings, and various forms of violence.

The poor—the 11–12 percent of the population with incomes still below the "poverty line,"[11] to whom good health habits are often an impossible luxury and who have historically suffered inadequate health care and inferior health status—were especially vulnerable during the inflationary sixties and early seventies. Not only is their discretionary income almost nil, but, thanks to television, advertising, and the general homogenization of middle-class values, they are expected to act as though they have the same purchasing power as the rich. Indeed, many younger males are enticed, practically as evidence of manhood, to try to acquire the purchasing power and the gratifications that advertisements dangle before them, by whatever means, legal or illegal, they can command.

THE INADEQUACY OF THERAPEUTIC MEDICINE

The results of these developments are evident in the nation's health statistics. Despite the vast increase in health care expenditures and greatly improved access to care on the part of most Americans, our status with respect to illness, disability, and premature death shows few—if any—signs of improvement. Polio and diphtheria-tetanus-pertussis (DTP) immunization rates for preschool children declined substantially, 1964-73.[12] By 1973 only 60.4 percent of the population had at least three doses of polio vaccine, and only 40.3 percent of the nonwhite youngsters in central cities. Preliminary data indicate a slight improvement in 1974, but there is now a potential for outbreaks of hitherto-controlled serious diseases.

Statistics with respect to death rates are particularly disturbing. After half a century of steady and dramatic improvement, the total or "crude" death rate for the United States ceased to improve during the sixties. Between 1960 and 1973 it remained almost stable, fluctuating between 9.7 and 9.3 per 1,000 population. The figure for 1973 is 9.4.[13] This stability, moreover, conceals a multitude of differential changes, some distinctly negative. For example:

- The stability of the total death rate in the sixties was primarily a function of changes in the population composition, not stable rates across time for all age groups.[14] When this effect is controlled, increases in the death rates for all age groups, 15–44, are revealed. Although there were some small increases for women, the increases were primarily for males, and the upturn was higher for blacks than for whites. This does not include battle deaths.[15]
- The sex differential in life expectancy is now greater than are race differentials. The female-male differential increased from one year in 1920 to 7.5 years in 1970.
- The age-adjusted death rate for homicide rose from 5.4 per 100,000 in 1950 to 10.5 in 1973 and seems destined to continue rising.[16]

The principal causes of death for the whole population in the late sixties were still the familiar trio—heart disease, cancer, and stroke, plus accidents.[17] In 1970 cardiovascular diseases accounted for 53 percent of all deaths. During the later sixties, however, other causes accounted for the rising death rates for young men. The principal cause of death for men, 15–44, was automobile accidents; homicide and suicide were also important.[18] None of these three phenomena is directly affected by the health care delivery system.

Death is, of course, the ultimate in poor health. It is also the best reported. But, it is only the tip of the iceberg. For every youngster killed in an automobile accident, hundreds are injured each year, many permanently disabled. For every middle-aged man who dies of cirrhosis, there are hundreds of alcoholics or near-alcoholics. For every death from an overdose of heroin, hundreds are hooked, perhaps for life, to a habit that will not only wreck their own lives but almost surely cause crime and other problems for their communities.

To many it appears that therapeutic medicine, important as it is, may have reached a point of diminishing returns. The 12–15 percent increases that we are adding to our $100 billion health care bill each year—even the portion that is not consumed by inflation—apparently have only a marginal utility.

This judgment relates not only to the large amount of preventable illness but to the shortcomings of medical intervention per se in the management of serious illness. Consider, for example, the widespread evidence of patient noncompliance with prescribed regimens; the growing evidence of unnecessary surgery[19] and overmedication;[20] the increasing realization that technical virtuosity is not necessarily synonymous with effective care;[21] the repeated exposés of miserable care in many nursing homes now expensively reimbursed under Medicare and Medicaid;[22] the growing public demand for more attention to the humanities and amenities of death and dying; and the renewed interest in euthanasia. All these developments indicate the public's growing impatience with overemphasis on the technology of medicine and neglect of the patient as a responsible agent in the treatment of his or her own illness.

The economist Victor Fuch's latest book, *Who Shall Live?*, provides scholarly documentation for this thesis. After comparing differences in health status among different groups in the United States, he points out,

> The most important thing to realize about such differences in health levels is that they are usually *not* related in any important degree to differences in medical care. Over time the introduction of new medical technology has had a significant impact on health, but when we examine differences among populations at a given moment in time, other socioeconomic and cultural variables are now much more important than differences in the quantity or quality of medical care.

To illustrate, Professor Fuchs develops his "tale of two states," Utah and Nevada:

> contiguous states that enjoy about the same levels of income and medical care and are alike in many other respects but their levels of health differ enormously. The inhabitants of Utah are among the healthiest individuals in the United States, while the residents of Nevada are at the opposite end of the spectrum. . . . What, then, explains these huge differences? . . . The answer almost surely lies in the different life styles of the residents of the two states.

As for efforts to improve the status of health in the United States, Fuchs concludes,

> The greatest current potential for improving the health of the American people is to be found in what they do or don't do to and for themselves. Individual decisions about diet, exercise, and smoking are of critical importance, and collective decisions affecting pollution and other aspects of the environment are also relevant.[23]

Proof of the Fuchs thesis was established several years ago by Dr. Lester Breslow, Dean of the School of Public Health, University of California at Los Angeles, and Dr. N. B. Belloc of the Human Population Laboratory, California State Department of Public Health, through a study of nearly seven thousand adults who were followed for five and one-half years. The results showed that life expectancy and better health are significantly related to a number of simple but basic health habits. These included:

1. three meals a day at regular times instead of snacks;
2. breakfast every day;
3. moderate exercise (long walks, bike riding, swimming, gardening) two or three times a week;
4. seven or eight hours sleep a night;
5. no smoking;
6. moderate weight;
7. no alcohol or only in moderation.

Among the specific findings:

1. A 45-year-old man who practices 0–3 of these habits has a life expectancy of 21.6 years; he can expect to live to about 67. A man with 6–7 of these habits can look forward to 33.1 years, to age 78. In the words of the author, "The magnitude of this difference of more than 11 years is better understood if we consider that the increase in the life expectancy of white men in the United States between 1900 and 1960 was only 3 years."
2. The physical health status of those reported following all seven good health practices was consistently about the same as those thirty years younger who followed few or none of these practices.[24]

The full impact of these facts has not yet permeated public thinking. Legislators, union leaders, and many segments of the health care establishment still speak as though the primary barrier to good health in America is lack of financial access. But the steam has gone out of this argument. Certainly there are many Americans who do not have access to quality care, and effective steps must be taken, through national health insurance and other means, to provide them with this access. Certainly there is need for improvement in the delivery of care, and in the education and distribution of health manpower.

The fact remains, however, that the primary cause of poor health and premature death in the United States today cannot be attributed either to lack of access or to shortcomings of the delivery system per se. In the words of a *New York Times* writer just returned from the village of Vilcabamba, Ecuador, noted for its centenarians, "Living a long life is essentially a do-it-yourself proposition."[25] The formal medical system merely patches up victims of heart attacks, automobile accidents, and attempted murder without usually affecting the underlying problems of poor diet, poor driving, or pent-up violence. A direct attack on the primary causes can only be made by efforts at prevention and education.

But this is not likely to happen automatically. For there is another important reason for the neglect of health education: lack of confidence in health education as an effective and reliable discipline. Even among health care sophisticates, who recognize the limits of therapeutic medicine and the crucial role of individual behavior and life style in the etiology of disease and disability in an affluent nation like ours, there is widespread skepticism as to the ability of health education to make any real difference. Indeed, there are some who say that health education today is nothing more than a slogan!

Others say this is much too strong an indictment; that thousands of dedicated men and women are working conscientiously in schools, local public health offices, neighborhood health centers, and other settings at jobs that bear the title "health educator," and hundreds more are preparing themselves for such careers at institutions of higher learning around the country. Obviously, there *is* a profession of health education.

Some critics attribute the alleged ineffectiveness to lack of knowledge as to how to bridge the gap between information and change in individual behavior; others cite the impossibility of effecting any meaningful change in the face of the overwhelming forces pressing in the opposite direction—pressing the individual to eat too much, drink too much, drive too fast, work too hard at sedentary jobs.

Part II addresses both these criticisms, reviewing current health education programs, practices, personnel, and problems—external as well as internal. It sets the stage for the recommendations in Part III.

Before undertaking this review, however, we look first at the rebirth of interest in health education and related activities, some important changes in the socioeconomic environment, and the new opportunities, as well as new obstacles, that these may present for reinvigoration of the profession and, possibly, even redefinition of the field.

A REBIRTH OF INTEREST IN HEALTH EDUCATION

Fortunately there now appears to be a renaissance of interest in prevention, health education, and increased consumer responsibility. Most striking is the plea from consumers themselves, who devour health information of all types. Witness the remarkable growth during the last few decades of do-it-yourself health literature, food stores, and related phenomena.

Part of the information disseminated in this way is worthless. Some is excellent, for example, the series of health information pamphlets published by the Public Affairs Committee, New York City, and the series, *Blue Print for Health*, published by the Blue Cross Association, Chicago. In either case, the public craving for information and guidance is genuine.

Physical fitness centers, commercial health spas, and active sports clubs of all types are springing up across the country. Concern among the young is growing.[26] Even sixth-graders write letters to their Congressional representatives pleading for environmental controls so they can live in a healthier world, and college students patronize health food restaurants and stores.

There is another dimension to consumer concern that goes beyond the desire for information or even better health. Individuals are demanding an active role in making policy for the health care system. Ralph Nader and the consumer movements have encouraged demands both for consumer participation in the decision-making processes of Blue Cross, hospital boards, and other health agencies, and for patients participation in medical decisions affecting their own lives and bodies. For example, the Boston Women's Health Collective prepared the book, *Our Bodies, Ourselves*,[27] to provide women with a basic understanding of the functioning of their bodies and to help them utilize the health care delivery system to their best advantage. The book met a need, not recognized by the traditional health system, and became a best seller on college campuses. Health cooperatives, neighborhood health centers, family-planning clinics, and other community-controlled programs have emphasized health information and education programs, often relying heavily on indigenous outreach workers.

There is also reason to believe that a substantial majority of the public feel the need for more information about health and medical care. A 1971 Harris survey, commissioned by the Blue Cross Association, reported that 56 percent felt such a need. Among blacks, persons under 30, and those with less than a college education, the percentage rose as high as 69 percent. Queried further as to desirable ways of disseminating information, the majority of respondents endorsed nine different sources of information. The largest vote—80 percent—went for "a system where health information is distributed by doctors and hospitals on a regular basis." Seventy-nine percent also approved clinics as sources of information, and 76 percent endorsed "better and more complete health care information on TV and radio."[28] A 1974 survey of 405 families in a typical middle-income community in central New Jersey found 61 percent interested in attending at least one formal health education program.[29]

Health professionals have responded to public, consumer, and patient concerns in many ways. For example:

- There is renewed interest in primary care and people-oriented specialties.

- Patient education, especially for those with chronic illness or disability, has been rediscovered in many hospitals and doctors' offices, and medical and hospital journals are devoting increasing attention to it.
- New theories and techniques of "behavior change"* are being developed by psychologists, psychiatrists, and others.
- The Blue Cross Association approved a special White Paper on Patient Health Education, not only endorsing the concept but urging third-party reimbursement therefor (see Appendix J).
- The American Hospital Association proclaimed patient education as one of its major priority items for 1974-75.[30]
- The plenary sessions of the Association of American Medical Colleges annual meeting in November 1974 focused entirely on public health education.[31]
- Some physicians and physician groups see patient education as an important bulwark against malpractice suits and the rising costs of malpractice insurance. Evidence of such interest varies from a panel on "Risk Control and Patient Education" at the National Conference on Medical Malpractice sponsored by the American Group Practice Association, March 1975, to the series of informational and risk-sharing booklets being developed on a business basis by a group of doctors in California.[32]

The growing interest on the part of consumers and providers has begun to be reflected at the federal level. One of the most impressive new initiatives has come from the National Institutes of Health. Both the National Cancer Institute and the National Heart and Lung Institute are currently funding consumer education and prevention programs that, according to an official spokesman, may now total $40–50 million dollars.[33]

In 1971 the prestigious President's Committee on Health Education was appointed. In 1973 the Health Insurance Benefits Advisory Council (HIBAC) to the Secretary of HEW established, for the first time, a Committee on Health Education, which helped to clarify Medicare and Medicaid reimbursement policies in this area. Publication of the President's Committee Report in 1973 provided a focus for national attention and led to two significant developments the following year: (1) establishment of a Bureau of Health Education in the Department of Health, Education, and Welfare's Center for Disease Control, and (2) an HEW contract with the National Health Council to prepare plans for establishment of a National Center for

---

*Although the term "behavior modification" is now widely used in the popular press to indicate almost any professionally directed effort to change individual behavior, the term as used by specialists generally implies a particular methodology. We have avoided use of the term in the broader, looser sense, substituting therefor the general phrase "behavior change."

Health Education "to stimulate, coordinate, and evaluate health education programs."[34]

Also in 1974 came three additional indications of growing government interest: (1) the first Congressional bill devoted exclusively to consumer health education was introduced by Representative Cohen of Maine (reintroduced in 1975 as H.R. 3205 with its companion bill, S. 1521, introduced by Senator Javits of New York); (2) public health education was listed as one of the ten national health priorities in the National Health Planning and Resources Development Act of 1974 (P.L. 93–641); and (3) the Department of Health, Education, and Welfare specified "a coherent set of health education initiatives" as one of the goals of its "Forward Plan for Health for FY 1976–1980."

In April 1975, just as this report was being completed, another and far more comprehensive health education bill was introduced into Congress by Congressman Carter of Kentucky and Senator Kennedy of Massachusetts (H.R. 5839 and S. 1467).

It is also worth noting that the renewed interest in consumer responsibility and health education is by no means only an American phenomenon. On the contrary, many other countries have historically paid far more attention to health education than we have. The Canadian experience is perhaps closer to ours. There, too, the emphasis in recent years has been almost entirely on therapeutic medicine. In 1974, however, the Minister of National Health and Welfare published an unusual document, *A New Perspective on the Health of Canadians*, which called for a reordering of national health priorities in favor of "health promotion" as opposed to "health care."[35] Implementation remains minimal, but the mere articulation of such a new policy at the highest level of government is significant.

Whether all this adds up to the beginning of a basic reorientation in the nation's health priorities, whether it presages a real and permanent revival of interest in health education, remains to be seen. It could be merely another passing fad, like many we have seen during the past two decades. It is still much too soon to be sure.

THE NEW ECONOMIC CLIMATE: CRISIS AND OPPORTUNITY

A major factor in the new climate of opinion is the radically changed economic picture, both national and international. In sharp contrast to the three previous decades, when real gross national product and real family income were rising consistently, both economic indicators are now falling. Along with the serious inflation, unemployment is also rising and, by early 1975 was well over 8 percent. International tensions, exacerbated by the growing shortages of food and fuel in a world once more haunted by the spectre of

Malthusian economics, dictate continued large expenditures on nonproductive armaments and impede international cooperation in the solution of our mutual concerns and problems.

What has all this to do with health education? It all depends on the definition and the concept of the role of health education in this new world of falling incomes and increasing shortages.

The President's Committee on Health Education defined health education as "a process that bridges the gap between health information and health practices." This definition is helpful in that it focuses attention on behavior change and points up the quintessential matter of motivation. However, it is doubtful that any amount of sophisticated psychological manipulation could have made up for the lack of motivation which, as we have seen, was so conspicuous in the sixties.

The current food, fuel, and general economic crises may present the most important stimulus for health education since World War II. What better time, for example, to publicize the harmful effects of too much sugar? too much marbleized beef? too many dairy products? To realize that the national diet can change one has only to note that in 1950 the average American ate 50 pounds of beef, and in 1973, 119 pounds.

Trying to get people to cut back on anything—sugar, cholesterol, or alcohol—is not easy. But it is possible. Fifty-two percent of the male population smoked cigarettes in 1966 two years after the Surgeon General issued his report on smoking and health; preliminary figures in 1970 indicate a decrease to 42 percent.[36] This is far from ideal, but apparently a change of even this relatively small magnitude has contributed to the dramatic recent reversal in the death rate from coronary heart disease. From 1950 to 1963, the age-adjusted death rate from this disease increased 19 percent. From 1963 to 1971 it fell 10.5 percent. In the words of the the cardiologist Weldon J. Walker, "Certainly, there can be a much greater future decline with more effective preventive and educational programs."[37]

But Dr. Walker does not rely on education or individual behavior change alone to bring about this "greater future decline." Accusing Congress of "using our tax money . . . to subsidize increased death and disability among our citizens," he calls for an end to federal price supports for tobacco and calls on organized medicine to "ask each individual seeking national elective office for a commitment to promptly correct this national shame."

Other physicians have called for higher taxes on cigarettes, the proceeds to be used for the care of individuals who have diseases related to smoking.[38] Dr. Walker's strong stand, coupled with an attack on the "Svengali psychologists of Madison Avenue," is endorsed editorially in the *Journal of the American Medical Association.*[39]

Dr. René Dubos, the distinguished scientist and author, has pointed out the possible benefits to health that could result from the current energy crisis:

> A recent study based on social indicators in 55 countries failed to reveal any beneficial effect of increased energy use on the quality of life. If there was a correlation, it was that the greater the energy consumption, the larger the percentage of divorces and suicides .... A decrease in energy use could have a multiplicity of beneficial effects in the long run. These would include improvements in physical and mental health .... The energy crisis will be a blessing if it compels us to develop ways of life that encourage fuller expression of the adaptive and creative potentialities that are present in us and in nature.[40]

Dr. Dubos' prediction has already proved partially correct. Accidents on the 142-mile New Jersey Turnpike dropped by one-fifth from 1973 to 1974, the first full year for the reduced speed limit, and fatalities were down by nearly half, to the lowest figure since 1966.[41]

According to the Chinese, the word "crisis" has two meanings—"danger" and "opportunity." The current world crises could perhaps provide the long-missing link, the motivation, to correct the destructive excesses of the American life style of the sixties, and to do it primarily through education and an appeal to intelligent self-interest rather than through government controls.

Can health education rise to the challenge?

Notes

1. U.S., Department of Health, Education, and Welfare, National Center for Health Statistics, *Monthly Vital Statistics Report—Summary Report Final Morbidity Statistics 1973*, February 10, 1975, table 6.

2. Ibid., table 3.

3. Ibid., table 6.

4. W. J. Walker, M.D., "Government Subsidized Death and Disability," *Journal of the American Medical Association*, December 16, 1974, p. 1530.

5. *New York Times*, November 12, 1974, citing an article in the *Lancet* by scientists at St. Thomas's Hospital and the London School of Hygiene and Tropical Medicine.

6. National Institute on Alcohol Abuse and Alcoholism, cited in "Alcoholism in the U.S.," *Statistical Bulletin* [Metropolitan Life], July 1974, p. 3.

7. Morris E. Chafetz, M.D., Director, National Institute on Alcohol Abuse and Alcoholism, *New York Times*, July 11, 1974.

8. *New York Times*, March 9, 1975.

9. U.S., Department of Health Education and Welfare, Social Security Administration, *Social Security Bulletin*, February 1976, p. 7.

10. President's Committee on Health Education, *Report*, Department of Health, Education, and Welfare, 1973, p. 25.

11. Assuming a minimum 1973 income of $4,540 for a family of four to be above the "poverty line," about 23 million, or 11 percent of the population, were below that level in that year, a considerable improvement over the past. The effect of the recent recession on this figure is not yet known. Dorothy Rice, Deputy Assistant Commissioner, Office of Research and Statistics, Social Security Administration, telephone communication, May 6, 1975.

12. U.S., Department of Health, Education, and Welfare, Center for Disease Control, Immunization Division, *Summary of Immunization Status for Polio, DTP, Measles, and Rubella, U.S., 1974*, Preliminary data from U.S. Immunization Survey, 1974, Atlanta, tables 1 and 7.

13. *Monthly Vital Statistics Report, . . . 1973*, table 4.

14. A. J. Klebba et al., *Mortality Trends: Age, Color, Sex, United States, 1950–69*, Department of Health, Education, and Welfare, National Center for Health Statistics, ser. 20, no. 15 (1973), pp. 3 ff.

15. More recent information from the National Center for Health Statistics indicates no change 1970–74 in the male death rate for ages 15–24, a slight improvement for ages 25–44. A. J. McDowell, Director, Division of Health Examination Statistics, National Center for Health Statistics, letter to chairman, April 28, 1975.

16. A. Joan Klebba, "Homicide Trends in the U.S., 1900–74," *Public Health Reports*, vol. 90, May–June 1975, table 2.

17. Some authorities would add alcohol-related deaths on the assumption that alcoholism is a major underlying factor in so much illness.

18. A. J. Klebba et al., *Leading Components of Upturn in Mortality for Men, United States, 1952–67*, Department of Health, Education, and Welfare, National Center for Health Statistics, ser. 20, no. 11 (1971). See also, A. J. Klebba et al., *Mortality Trends for Leading Causes of Death, U.S. 1950–69*, Department of Health, Education, and Welfare, National Center for Health Statistics, ser. 20, no. 16 (1974).

19. E.g., E. G. McCarthy, M.D. and G. W. Widmer, R.N., "Effects of Screening by Consultants on Recommended Elective Surgical Procedures," *New England Journal of Medicine*, December 19, 1974, pp. 1331–35.

20. U.S., Congress, Senate, Special Committee on Aging, Subcommittee on Long-term Care, *Nursing Home Care in the U.S.: Failure in Public Policy*, supporting paper no. 2: *Drugs in Nursing Homes: Misuse, High Costs and Kickbacks*, 94th Cong., 1st sess., January 1975. According to this source, "20 to 40 percent of nursing home drugs are administered in error." (p. xi).

21. E.g., F. J. Cook, "The Operation Was a Success But the Patient Died," *New York Magazine*, vol. 7, no. 46, November 18, 1974, pp. 121–151.

22. E.g., Senate Special Committee on Aging, *Nursing Home Care in the U.S. Introductory Report*, et seq.; New York Temporary Commission on Living Costs and the Economy (Stein Commission), reports *New York Times, January–March 1975.

23. V. R. Fuchs, *Who Shall Live? Health, Economics, and Social Choice* (New York; Basic Books, 1974), p. 16, 52–55.

24. L. Breslow, M.D., "A Quantitative Approach to the World Health Organization Definition of Health," *International Journal of Epidemiology*, vol. 1. no. 4, Winter 1972, pp. 347–55; N. B. Belloc and L. Breslow, "Relationship of Physical Health Status and Health Practices," *Preventive Medicine*, vol. 1, no. 3, August 1972, pp. 409–21; N. B. Belloc, "Relationship of Health Practices and Mortality," *Preventive Medicine*, vol. 2, 1973, pp. 67–81.

25. Grace Halsell, *New York Times*, March 1, 1975, Op. Ed. page. There is, of course, a danger that this point of view, like its opposite, can be carried too far and lead to a new form of medical

nihilism. See, for example, Ivan Illich, *Medical Nemesis: The Expropriation of Health* (London: Calder and Boyars, Ltd., 1975).

26. Transcendental meditation, a technique of inducing deep relaxation that has been reported to result in significant physiological as well as behavioral changes, is now spreading rapidly not only on college campuses but in various health care settings. Even if reports of reduced smoking, drug abuse, and drinking and of lowered blood pressure are exaggerated, the motivation of those seeking such assistance is important and relevant to the concerns of the Task Force. See M. Scarf, "Tuning Down with TM," *New York Times Magazine*, February 9, 1975, pp. 12 ff.; G. Williams, "Sit Back, Close Your Eyes, Turn Off . . . ," *Science Digest*, vol. 76, no. 5., November 1974, pp. 70–75.

27. Boston Women's Health Book Collective, *Our Bodies, Ourselves* (New York: Simon and Schuster, 1973).

28. Blue Cross Association, "Harris Study Stresses Health Education Need," press release, Chicago, December 29, 1971, pp. 18–19.

29. P. Vasilenko, "East Brunswick Township Health Needs Survey," Princeton University Woodrow Wilson School, term paper, January 1975 (processed), p. 28. The greatest demand was for courses on heart disease/hypertension; the smallest for V.D.

30. American Hospital Association, *Statement on the Role and Responsibilities of Hospitals and Other Health Care Institutions in Personal and Community Health Education* (Chicago: American Hospital Association, 1974).

31. See articles by Governor Terry Sanford; W. J. McNerney; H. J. Barnum, Jr.; D. C. Tosteson, M.D.; A. M. Schmidt, M.D.; Governor D. J. Evans; Secretary C. W. Weinberger; and W. H. Kobin in the *Journal of Medical Education*, January and February 1975.

32. *DocuBooks* (San Diego: Health Com-Health Communications, Inc). The booklets, relating primarily to various surgical procedures, come with or without a legal "informed consent" form at the back.

33. Harrison Owen, Program Coordinator, Office of Prevention, Control, and Education, National Heart and Lung Institute, letter to chairman, January 21, 1975.

34. President's Committee on Health Education, *Report*, p. 28.

35. Mark Lalonde, *A New Perspective on the Health of Canadians*, Ministry of National Health and Welfare, Ottawa, 1974. See also, A. R. Somers, "Recharting National Health Priorities: A New Canadian Perspective," *New England Journal of Medicine*, August 22, 1974, pp. 415–16.

36. U.S., Department of Health, Education, and Welfare, Center for Disease Control, National Clearinghouse for Smoking and Health, *Adult Use of Tobacco*, DHEW Publ. (HSM) 73–8727, Atlanta, June 1973.

37. Walker, "Government Subsidized Death and Disability," p. 1530. See also, Jeremiah B. Stamler, M.D., cited in J. E. Brody, "Drop Reported in Coronary Death Rate," *New York Times*, January 24, 1975.

38. Leroy Schwartz, M.D., interview, Princeton, January 19, 1975.

39. R. H. Moser, M.D., "The New Seduction," *Journal of the American Medical Association*, December 16, 1974, p. 1564.

40. René Dubos, "Less Energy, Better Life," *New York Times*, January 7, 1975, Op. Ed. page.

41. *New York Times*, February 23, 1975.

Part II
Current Programs, Practices, and Major Problems

DEFINITIONS, GOALS, AND NATIONAL POLICY

Here are some current definitions of "health education":

- "Health education is guiding individuals or groups to perceive given healthful actions as being in line with their own values and goals."[1]
- "Health education is an integral part of high-quality health care . . . . The major emphasis . . . is health promotion, which includes health maintenance, disease and trauma management, and the improvement of the health care system and its utilization."[2]
- " 'Health education' . . . may be defined as the process of providing learning experiences which favorably influence understandings, attitudes, and conduct in regard to individual and community health."[3]
- "Health education is a process that bridges the gap between health information and health practices."[4]
- "The ultimate goal of health education is the improvement of the nation's health and the reduction of preventable illness, disability, and death . . . . Health education is that dimension of health care that is concerned with influencing behavioral factors."[5]
- "The objectives of health education are:

  (1) to improve the health of the people . . . by (a) providing them the necessary information to help prevent illness and disability insofar as possible and to maintain the highest possible level of well-being even when ill or disabled; and (b) helping them to make the necessary modification in individual life style or behavior when necessary;

  (2) to help restrain inflation in health care costs by relieving some of the preventable demand on health services;

  (3) to involve the consumer/patient positively and constructively in his own health maintenance and in responsible effective use of the health care delivery system."[6]

15

The common factors in these attempts at definition are obvious: the concern with prevention of illness and disability and the emphasis on influencing individual behavior. Beyond these elements of agreement, however, there are many important differences and inconsistencies. For example:

• Is health education a subdivision of health care? Or a separate category of activity? Or sometimes one and sometimes the other?

• Is health education synonymous with health promotion? If not, how should each term be defined? What is the major distinction?

• Is health education provided primarily by means of a series of structured "learning experiences"? Or is it any activity that guides individuals or groups toward more healthful actions?

• Does health education start where health information leaves off and stop where health policy begins? Or is it a combination of two of these? Or all three?

• Does health education aim primarily at the adjustment of individual behavior in the face of health-threatening external forces? Or at the adjustment of these forces? Or both?

These are not merely academic questions. They suggest one reason for the vast discrepancy between the lofty goals frequently advanced by advocates of health education and the limited achievements. They also suggest the difficulty of defining meaningful professional or national policy in this area.

For example, if health education is, as the American Hospital Association states, an "integral part of high-quality health care," why is it that only a handful of the nation's seven thousand hospitals maintain even a token health education program and that only a handful of the nation's health education specialists are employed in any part of the health care delivery system?

If the National Education Association and the American Medical Association believe that health education is a process that "favorably influences understandings, attitudes, and conduct in regard to individual and community health," how is it that most of the nation's schools continue to support programs that conspicuously fail to do these things?

At the national level the inconsistency becomes compounded. In his opening address to the Conference on Health Education sponsored by the Center for Disease Control's new Bureau of Health Education in June 1974, Dr. Charles Edwards, former Assistant Secretary for Health, proclaimed this broad and lofty goal for health education:

> Success in health education . . . has to be measured in human
> terms—lives saved, suffering and disability reduced, productivity
> and creativity enhanced, and something called the quality of life
> made more rewarding for everyone. That sounds like a tall order to

lay at the doorstep of health education. And, certainly, it is, but, realistically, how could we be satisfied with less?[7]

To fulfill this "tall order" the bureau was budgeted $3.5 million for FY 1975,[8] most of which was merely transferred from existing programs. Queried as to its budget request for 1976, Mr. Horace Ogden, Director of the Bureau, replied, "About $4 million."[9] These figures may be compared with the total federal health budget for 1975 of $26.3 billion.[10]

Granted that the federal government is actually spending much more for health education than the bureau budget suggests (see, for example, Part I, p. 9), the fact remains that this is the office singled out by the Administration, with the approval of Congress, to develop and carry out health education policy for the entire federal health establishment. Faced with such discrepancy between the rhetoric and the reality, we can only conclude that there is no meaningful national policy on health education today.

Indeed, we go further and say there is no national policy on health promotion. The rhetoric is there, in full measure. But when the claims of the public health are weighed against the claims of other, better-organized or more articulate interests, the latter generally prevail. A dramatic example comes from the juxtaposition of the Administration's "Forward Plan for Health for FY 1976–1980," with the Medicare law, the nation's principal instrument for financial support of health care. While the former proclaims "prevention" as priority number one, the latter prohibits reimbursement for preventive care.

Other examples of inconsistent federal policies in this area abound. For example:

• The National Heart and Lung Institute was allocated $175 million for research in heart and vascular diseases in 1975.[11] At the same time, the U.S. Department of Agriculture placed its highest seal of approval— "prime"—on marbleized beef with a high fat content, thought by most cardiologists and nutritionists to contribute to high cholesterol levels, a major risk factor in heart disease.

• The Law Enforcement Assistance Administration distributed in 1975 an estimated $774 million in block grants to state and local governments for crime prevention, increased police protection, and other components of the criminal justice system.[12] Yet Congress has repeatedly refused to enact gun control legislation that could help to reduce homicide and other crime rates.

• A fourth of the children examined under the Medicaid Early Periodic Screening and Detection Program have needed dental care.[13] Sweets are a major factor in the incidence of dental caries. Yet the 1975 federal budget includes $91.5 million for payments to growers for producing sugar under the U.S. Sugar Act.[14]

• The U.S. Surgeon General determined, in 1964, that cigarette smoking is hazardous to health. Yet the Department of Agriculture continues to encourage tobacco production though price support, export programs, tobacco grading, and other services for farmers.[15]

By and large, health educators have ignored these broad policy issues. As a result, they have been working under almost insuperable handicaps. Concentrating almost exclusively on individual behavior adjustment while ignoring the overwhelming external pressures in the other direction can only be self-defeating.

Dr. Scott K. Simonds, who is a member of this Task Force, and a few other leaders of the profession have tried to influence health education to become more policy oriented and far broader, both in policy and application, than in the past.[16] For an excellent statement of this view, see Appendix C. The Task Force is in full agreement.

There is also a danger, however, in pushing this view too far. Overemphasis on broad policy issues to the neglect of more traditional individual instruction could lead to loss of identity for health education as a profession.

This, in our view, would also be unfortunate. What is needed is balance, a balance that we have tried to maintain throughout this report and in our recommendations. But if health education is to survive as a profession, rather than just a movement or a philosophy of life, it must acquire more precise discipline. This, in turn, calls for more precise definition of both goals and methodology.

CLASSIFICATION OF PROGRAMS

The large and confusing variety of programs that identify themselves, or could be identified, as "health education" almost defy logical classification. There is no accepted typology in this field. The following attempt is based on the institutional setting of the program and/or the primary target audience.

The brief descriptions that follow are for illustrative purpose only. They do not pretend to provide a comprehensive summary of activities under any of the six categories.

1. Patient Education in Hospitals and Other Health Care Institutions

A consumer becomes a patient when he or she recognizes a health problem or a potential problem and turns to a physician, clinic, hospital, or some other component of the health care delivery system for assistance. This distinction between consumer and patient is important. Patients have recognized a problem and made a commitment of time and frequently of money. They are, therefore, presumably more receptive to medical intervention and health education efforts.

However, recent studies of patient compliance with therapeutic regimens indicate a surprisingly large gap between what the doctor prescribes and what the patient does. For example, a study of patients with congestive heart failure (CHF) found that only slightly over half took their digitalis as prescribed.[17] Dr. T. F. Williams, University of Rochester School of Medicine, recently summarized the results of a number of studies of diabetes patient compliance with recommended measures as to diet, medications, urine testing, and foot care, and came to the following conclusion: "Overall, less than 10 percent of the patients observed were carrying out a minimally adequate regimen in all of these areas of day-to-day management of their diabetes."[18]

A summary of the magnitude of compliance with medications for cure of various conditions indicates a mean of about 50 percent with a huge variance. About one-third always comply, one-third never comply, and one-third sometimes.[19]

The authors of the CHF study concluded,

> The reliability of self-medication is related to understanding of the pathological process. . . . Patients who did not understand their illness told the interviewer that their physicians either did not tell them about their disease or, if they did, that their explanation was too technical. . . . There are obvious communication difficulties. These difficulties may relate in part to education which has been shown to affect patient compliance in other studies. In our study, 20 of 27 patients (75 percent) with an eighth-grade education or more took digitalis as often as prescribed compared to 13 of 33 (39 percent) who were less well educated.[20]

The implications both for general education and patient education are clear.

A large proportion of patient education is done on an informal one-to-one basis by physicians in their own offices, by nurses, therapists, and other health professionals. They are usually under severe time constraints and cannot provide either in-depth coverage of the instructional material or follow-up. The quality and content vary widely.

Organized classes and courses, usually for groups of patients referred by their doctor or nurse, are becoming more common. A considerable body of literature on the subject has appeared in recent years, most of it merely descriptive of individual programs with very little evaluation.

The American Hospital Association (AHA), as already noted, and several state hospital associations have taken a strong position in favor of hospital-based patient education. The AHA maintains a small staff of health educators and holds periodic conferences and workshops on the subject.[21] Despite this encouragement, only a small number of hospitals have established formal programs. The obstacles are great, involving lack of funds, inadequate patient demand, and very important, frequent lack of support from the medical and nursing staffs.

The formal programs in those hospitals that have them have usually been started through one of three types of activities: classes for diabetics, cardiac patients, or others with serious chronic diseases or disability; classes for expectant parents; and preoperative instruction. For each of these categories there is a large potential "student body," and the information and procedures are fairly well established. Instruction is usually provided upon referral by a doctor or nurse, on a group basis, and by a member of the professional staff.

Appendix D provides an illustrative list of patient education classes provided in a medium-sized community hospital in Trenton, New Jersey, during 1974. This hospital's commitment goes beyond teaching assorted courses: it has a full-time health education coordinator to identify problem areas, gather resources, and coordinate ongoing efforts. It also assumes responsibility for teaching the teachers; most of the "inservice programs" are directed at nurses.

Some health maintenance organizations (HMOs) and clinics are also operating formal health education programs.[22] For many years, the Health Insurance Plan of Greater New York (HIP) has been operating a large-scale educational program, until recently under the guidance of Dr. Irving S. Shapiro, a member of this Task Force. Several of the Kaiser-Permanente units operate health education activities; in the Oakland program there is extensive use of audiovisual equipment. The 1973 requirement that, to be eligible for federal financial funding, an HMO must provide "education in the contribution each member can make to the maintenance of his own health,"[23] has led to renewed interest in the subject.[24]

A few state and local health departments are active in this respect. The Veterans Administration, which issued its first policy statement on patient education as early as 1953, has recently initiated a major new program, placing patient education coordinators in each of its regions. In North Carolina, for example, the University of North Carolina School of Public Health is working with seven VA hospitals in that region.

There is an obvious chicken-and-egg relationship between the growth of patient education programs and the development of new hardware and software for teaching such programs. Several of the larger and more imaginative drug companies and appliance manufacturers have entered the field with films, tapes, cassettes, slides, anatomical models, teaching texts, and other audiovisual and printed teaching aids. Some are very good; most are expensive. One of the most interesting is the extensive program developed by Core Communications in Health, partly owned by Warner-Lambert Company, which is now being tried out in several clinics affiliated with the American Group Practice Association.[25]

A related development is the acquisition of several successful behavior change programs by large commercial enterprises, e.g., Weight Watchers, Incorporated by Pillsbury Flour Company, and Smoke-Enders by Schick Manufacturing Corporation. For-profit development of health education and behavior change programs can be useful; obviously, there is also substantial potential for abuse.

Although not strictly health education, the Health Hazard Appraisal Program developed at Methodist Hospital, Indianapolis,[26] is an important tool for alerting the asymptomatic to potential dangers and, it is hoped, for motivating them toward health education.

Despite the excellence of some of the new patient programs, in general the field of patient education lacks defined goals and methodologies, for both teaching and evaluation, as well as reliable sources of financing (see below). The diabetologists, under leadership of the American Diabetes Association, have probably come closer to standardized concepts and procedures than any other medical specialty. See, for example, the statement on "Health Education in the Primary Care Setting," Appendix E. An interdisciplinary American Association of Diabetes Educators has been established, with membership including physicians, nurses, dietitians, and others. The American Heart Association and American Cancer Society have played strong leadership roles in their respective areas.

Following are some of the more innovative recent approaches to patient education:

- the professional-patient "contract" developed by a group of leading diabetologists primarily as a stimulus and guide to patient motivation,[27] now being studied by physicians dealing with other chronic diseases;
- the "Activated Patient" course offered by Georgetown University's Community Health Plan at Reston, Virginia;[28]
- behavior modification programs for the obese developed in the Stanford University School of Medicine, Department of Psychiatry;[29]
- a "systems approach" to the planning, development, and design of a large consumer health education program is presented in a new handbook published by U.S. Army–Baylor University Program in Health Care Administration.[30]

Development of disease-specific, clinically tested teaching and evaluation protocols are essential prerequisites to third-party reimbursement, accreditation by the Joint Commission on the Accreditation of Hospitals (JCAH), and/or evaluation by Professional Standards Review Organizations (PSROs).

2.   School Health Education

The school, as a social structure, provides an educational setting in which the total health of the child during the impressionable years is of priority concern. No other community setting even approximates the magnitude of the grades K–12 school educational enterprise, with an enrollment in 1973–74 of 45.5 million in nearly 17,000 school districts comprising more than 115,000 schools with some 2.1 million teachers. . . . Additionally, more than 40 percent of children aged three to five are enrolled in early childhood education programs. Thus, it seems that the school should be regarded as a social unit providing a focal point to which health planning for all other community settings should relate.[31]

This forceful statement by the American Public Health Association emphasizes the magnitude of the virtually "captive" audience for school health education and the resources available for reaching that audience. The urgency of reaching it with meaningful health education has become clearer as we begin to understand more fully the pathological, as well as the psychological, meaning of the concept William Wordsworth expressed poetically, "The child is father of the man."

For example, Drs. Blumenthal and Jesse of the University of Miami School of Medicine tell us, "If intervention to modify coronary risk factors is put off till adulthood, it may well prove ineffective. Pathologic studies have shown that by the third decade many Americans have already advanced lesions in the aorta and the coronary arteries."[32] For discussion of the importance of good nutrition education in the schools as well as later in life, see Appendix O by Task Force member, Barbara E. Anlyan.

Unfortunately, there is very little evidence that either the challenge or the opportunity inherent in school health education has even been appreciated, much less acted on. On the contrary, even overt health problems, such as care of the diabetic school child, are frequently neglected.[33]

Both the quantity and quality of health education efforts vary widely across school districts: in some it is an integral part of the education process; in others it is merely a substitute for gym on a rainy day; in still others, it is not available at all. In general, the record is poor.[34]

It is difficult to determine which states have effective school health education programs. Many have enacted legislation or issued administrative directives mandating health education in public schools. Frequently, however, funds have not been appropriated to implement and enforce these regulations.

Recently several states have adopted comprehensive school health education requirements, covering all grades from kindergarten to 12 and encouraging coverage of a wide range of topics. New York, which passed legislation in the mid-sixties, was the first to adopt such requirements, and it has backed its legislation with both funding and enforcement. Since 1972 Illinois, Iowa, Florida, Michigan, Oklahoma, and New Mexico have followed suit, although Florida and Michigan have not yet allocated funds.[35]

School health education programs are faced with three major constraints: (a) a tradition of low visibility and low priority, (b) a narrow definition of the appropriate content and jurisdiction for health education efforts, and (c) a shortage of adequately trained health educators.

School administrators and school boards are frequently unaware of the importance of health education, and there is no enforcement power within school systems to ensure that health education is actually provided. Health education is frequently tacked on to another department and can be found buried in home economics, biology, or physical education. It is often not separately delineated in school budgets. Therefore, realistic assessments of the resources allocated for school health education are not available. Without departments or even faculty members to represent it, the low visibility continues.

Second, the content of health education in the past was often limited to dry discussions of hygiene and/or moralistic treatment of sex, drugs, and alcohol. This approach often engendered resistance and resentment. In recent years this orientation has begun to change; healthful behavior is treated as a positive force in the students' lives. This change is reflected at the secondary level by courses in family living taught in home economics departments and by training in "lifetime" sports such as tennis, swimming, and golf in physical education departments. At the elementary level, teachers are integrating health education into ongoing reading and science classes and developing special health education programs.

The shortcomings of curricula are still substantial. Open discussions of sex, contraception, drug use and abuse—subjects of immediate concern to many teenagers—are often barred from the classroom by political constraints and tradition. Discussions of how to use the fragmented health care delivery system are usually not included at all. Such information is particularly important for blacks, Chicanos, Puerto Ricans, and the poor, who are often excluded from the traditional health care system and must maneuver their way through the red tape of Medicaid and clinic programs. Textbooks written for white, middle-class students, which admonish them to eat meat daily or to see their doctor if certain symptoms appear, are also not relevant to these groups.

Health education to inform youngsters on anatomy and physiology, where available, appears to be acceptable and effective. Education to influence behavior, by contrast, is largely a dream for the future. Indeed, there are reports to indicate that teaching children about alcohol, drugs, sex, and even driving may have adverse effects. It may be that, for some of the young, ignorance is blissfully beneficial since familiarity often breeds contempt.

The adolescents most in health jeopardy are those least likely to behave in accord with facts and logic and most likely to be attracted toward actions perceived as dangerous or actually disapproved. They are to be found most often among school dropouts and, hence, are not even in the classroom when health presentations are made.

Research is needed to determine the best techniques for influencing adolescent conformity and peer acceptance, the most important molders of behavior in those years when health habits are fixed. Even the optimum ages for introducing health information have not yet been determined.

An imaginative large-scale experiment in providing health education to economically disadvantaged young men and women, 16–21, was developed by the Job Corps at its sixty-five residential centers across the nation. Some 45,000–50,000 young people have been going through the centers annually and receiving ten to thirty hours of required health education.[36]

Another significant experiment, developed primarily by Dr. Carter Marshall, a member of this Task Force, is the Student Health Opportunities Program (SHOP), now known as Secondary Education Through Health (SETH), operated by the Mount Sinai School of Medicine, Department of Community Medicine, in New York City. Aimed at both health education and recruitment of minority students for the health professions, the program has operated in one of Manhattan's largest high schools, a school with an overall dropout rate of about 70 percent. After six years, dropouts from SHOP have averaged less than 5 percent. All eighty-five SHOP seniors in the class of 1975 graduated, and 90 percent went on to college with plans to pursue a health career.[37]

A research program with tremendous potential for future school health education is being conducted at the University of California in Los Angeles by Dr. Charles Lewis, Department of Medicine, and Mary Ann Lewis, University Elementary School. Starting with a study of the impact of television commercials on preschool age children,[38] Dr. and Mrs. Lewis have become convinced of the importance of the child as a decision maker and participant in sharing authority and responsibility for his own care.[39]

The third shortcoming—a shortage of school health educators —is related to the two just discussed. The shortage is both quantitative and qualitative. The number of professional school health educators is small; a maximum of

10,500 can be identified.[40] The other classroom teachers who assume responsibility for health education have little or no specialized training in the subject.

The training of school health educators varies from state to state. A 1968 survey revealed that only twenty-five of the forty-five responding states recognize both a major or minor in health education and require secondary school teachers to teach only subjects for which they have completed a major or minor. At the elementary school level, teachers are not usually required to specialize in a subject area. Within these guidelines. separate school districts often establish their own requirements, Although teacher certification is not needed to teach a particular subject in many of the states, forty-three responding states have established teacher certification procedures in health education. Reflecting a growing trend toward separating health education and physical education programs, eight states certify health educators separately. Fifteen, however, still combine the two fields, and twenty additional states provide an option. The course content of certification programs is varied, Only twelve states demand credits in health content, and in Missouri only two credits are required.[41]

Several programs have been initiated to expand the capabilities of general classroom instructors. The Berkeley Project, sponsored by the National Clearinghouse for Smoking and Health, teaches specific curricula for grades 4, 5, 6, and 8 to teams from individual school districts. The team consists of two teachers of the same grade, the administrator, and one or two auxiliary health professionals. The team then becomes the core trainer group for other teachers of the same grade level.[42]

Other school districts have expanded their capacities by hiring health educators to develop and coordinate programs throughout the school system; one example is the Arlington, Massachusetts, public school system.

In a unique effort to bridge the usual gulf between school health educators and health care professionals, the College of Medicine and Dentistry of New Jersey, Office of Consumer Health Education and Monmouth Medical Center, Long Branch, New Jersey, jointly sponsored a six-week summer health education project for 12-year-olds, July-August 1974, at a school in nearby Rumson. Young medical, nursing, and other health profession students were the instructors.[43]

Federal legislation to make health education a vital component of all public school programs has been proposed. Representative Lloyd Meeds of Washington, with fifty cosponsors, and Senator Richard Clark of Iowa, with six cosponsors, have introduced identical bills (H.R. 2599 and S. 544) to provide teacher training, pilot and demonstration projects, and grants to state and local educational agencies for development of comprehensive elementary and secondary school health programs. The three-year proposal, known as the Comprehensive School Health Education Act, would authorize up to $140 million for these three types of programs. Hearings were held in the House of Representatives in March 1975.

Institutions of higher education, no less than secondary and elementary schools, should be concerned with health education, both for their own students and the general public. Their past record in both respects has been undistinguished. There are hopeful signs, however. The responsibility is beginning to be recognized.[44] The American College Health Association is seriously addressing the problem of student health education, and the results are already obvious in the new orientation of many student health services. The revolution in sex education is particularly conspicuous.[45]

3. Occupational Health Education

Individuals are exposed to environmental hazards in their place of work that can have severe implications for their health. The Occupational Safety and Health Administration (OSHA) identifies two categories of risk: (1) safety hazards or dangerous physical conditions such as inadequate guards on machines; and (2) health hazards or unsafe levels of toxic substances and harmful physical agents such as asbestos and carbon monoxide.

Over the years, great progress has been made in reducing occupational safety and health hazards affecting American workers.[46] It has been pointed out that for every industrial accident death there are now fifty cardiovascular casualties.[47] In a dynamic technological society such as ours, however, new hazards constantly arise and old ones reappear in new forms. Some employers are still resistant to government or union-inspired efforts to control toxic substances. The Task Force heard several dramatic examples from a spokesman for the Health Research Group, a Nader-assisted public interest organization.[48]

To detect and control new hazards and to inculcate in the employee better understanding of his own responsibilities, as well as rights, under the federal occupational safety and health laws, OSHA has undertaken an extensive employee educational program. Employees can obviously affect the safety of their environment by following recognized safety practices such as wearing hard hats and ear plugs. However, in the more subtle area of health hazards, which are often difficult to detect without sophisticated equipment, their only protection often is knowing and acting on their legal rights. They can also request OSHA inspections when they suspect a hazardous health condition exists (and have their names withheld from their employers), and they can review their employers' records for monitoring and measuring hazardous materials.

In fiscal years 1974 and 1975, OSHA allocated $6.6 million for fifteen grants related to health education projects that test models of occupational health education.[49] The formats and curricula OSHA obtains from these projects can be adapted by employees and employee groups to their own particular needs. A substantial multiplier effect is anticipated.

The largest contract, for $3 million, was let to the National Safety Council, which has developed four short courses and implemented them through thirty-nine participating local safety councils. The courses include orientation to rights and responsibilities under the act and instructions on setting up safety and health programs within establishments. Over 100,000 individuals have already been reached by this massive, geographically dispersed program. Another contract demonstrates the feasibility of using community and junior colleges as part of the job safety and health education delivery system, while a third entails the creation of thirty-minute television programs on selected job safety and health topics.[50]

Training individuals to recognize health hazards is complex because the problems vary by occupation. OSHA has selected five "target industries" in which the disability and death rates are substantially above average: longshoring, meat and meat products, roofing and sheet metal, lumber and wood products, and miscellaneous transportation equipment.

OSHA's work has been supplemented by that of a number of unions and companies which have initiated their own education programs in areas not related to occupational safety but using the workplace as a focus for more general health education. For example, the United Mine Workers Union, which administers its own prepaid health insurance plan, has hired full-time health educators in several regions and conducts programs in preventive care and specialized classes for diabetics and others.[51]

The Connecticut Mutual Life Insurance Company in Hartford, Connecticut, and the Scoville Manufacturing Company in Waterbury, Connecticut, have programs to help workers with alcohol or other drug problems. In addition, Connecticut Mutual offers employees periodic voluntary physical examinations, occasional videotape presentations during the lunch hour on topics such as heart disease or alcoholism, and frequent health articles in company publications.[52]

The programs of both companies direct their promotional efforts largely toward supervisory personnel in the hope that they will refer workers who appear to have problems. Because of the savings resulting from increased worker output, Scoville no longer considers its program a cost item. In fact, savings in the Waterbury plant alone, which employs about 4,000 of the company's 24,000 workers nationwide, are estimated to be more than $200,-000 for 1974.[53]

Annual health examinations and counseling programs for executives, periodic screening of blue-collar employees, lunch-hour lectures on a variety of health topics for both blue-collar and white-collar workers: these and many other general health maintenance and educational activities are currently taking place throughout American business and industry. Such efforts, successful as they have proved to be in individual situations, have scarcely made a dent in the general health problems of American workers. The blame, however, cannot be attributed primarily either to management or the unions. The major culprits are the same four that hamper other forms of health education—individual ignorance, public apathy, commercial pressures, and lack of any strong, positive leadership on the part of either the government or the health professions.

4. Community Health Education

Categories 4 and 5—community programs and general or national programs—obviously overlap, and a strong case could be made for combining them. They have been separated here because of significant differences in scale, sponsorship, personnel, financing, and methodologies.

Community programs tend to be much smaller and localized. They are usually sponsored by a hospital, local health or welfare body, the "Y," or some other community group. They also tend to be directed toward defined populations, identified on the basis of geographic, socioeconomic, ethnic, age, or other factors.

Where programs are sponsored by a hospital, there may be an unbroken continuum of those designed for asymptomatic community groups, ambulatory patients, and inpatients. Frequently, the same personnel are involved. Third-party financing, however, is generally not available for community programs, and other public and private funds are usually available only on a demonstration basis. There is an urgent need to strengthen and make more systematic the financing of community programs.

The goal of targeted community programs is to identify individuals who are at risk, make them aware of the risk and of the steps they can take to reduce that risk, and, if symptoms are brought to light, to direct them to the appropriate care setting. Targeted community programs frequently start with screening—for hypertension, tuberculosis, breast cancer, sickle cell anemia, and so forth. Immediately after Mrs. Ford's and Mrs. Rockefeller's cancer operations, many communities throughout the nation rushed to set up cancer screening programs and classes in breast self-examination.

The value of many of the community programs, including "health fairs" and screening, is widely questioned. The latter can be evaluated either as a case-finding device or as an educational tool; the two are not necessarily the same. Debates about multiphasic screening, for example—whether it is an essential device in prevention or a poor use of money and an intrusion into the physician-patient relationship[54]—have occurred for twenty-five years without producing a consensus. Only recently have preliminary results from a randomized, controlled evaluation become available. The results from a study begun in 1964 by the Kaiser-Permanente Medical Care Program indicate that screening can reduce the number of "potentially postponable" deaths[55] and reduce medical costs for older men by $800 a year.[56]

A major problem in all screening is the difficulty of obtaining follow-up compliance. Forty thousand employed individuals potentially at risk for heart trouble were screened by the Chicago Chapter of the American Heart Association in 1967; over half scored too high on at least one of the three risk factors. The association sent up to three letters to encourage a professional visit, but the follow-up rate was still poor.[57]

Despite the inconclusive results of many screening programs, authoritative opinion is now on the side of clear, albeit cautious, endorsement. The educational potential is widely acknowledged. The National Academy of Sciences—National Research Council has just completed a major study, portions of which are included in a summary pamphlet, *Genetic Screening: Procedural Guidance and Recommendations*. The first recommendation states, "Genetic screening, when carried out under controlled conditions, is an appropriate form of medical care when the following criteria are met." Among the criteria are that "appropriate public education can be carried out" and that "education is effective." The indispensable link between effective screening and effective education is discussed in some detail.[58]

The informational "hot line" is another approach to community education that has been successfully used in some communities. At Monmouth Medical Center in Long Branch, New Jersey, a VD hot line increased the number of VD visits substantially and directed callers away from the hospital emergency room to the less costly clinic.[59]

Hot lines can also be operated on a community-wide basis and provide general (nonspecific) information on a variety of health and related topics. An alleged advantage of the hot line is that it is strictly informational. Callers can do what they wish with the information—use it or ignore it—and thus feel less threatened by professional manipulation. The opposite side of the coin is that much of the information is wasted.

In many low-income communities the usual difficulties confronting health education are compounded by cultural and other factors interfering with effective communication between providers and consumers. In Los Angeles, Detroit, Brooklyn, Durham, North Carolina, Trenton, New Jersey, and elsewhere, programs utilizing indigenous health education aides, "facilitators," outreach workers, or others with similar titles are currently in progress or under development. In the words of one sponsor,

> The principal difference between the Community Health Facilitator Program and a more conventional health education approach, is the emphasis that the [former] . . . places on the use of the existing strengths of a target community. . . . Although many agencies

and groups see as a first step to action the organization of the community, we feel it is more important to first look at how the community has already organized itself and then capitalize on and strengthen this existing organization.[60]

There is, as we see it, no inherent conflict between the indigenous community aide and the more highly trained professional. Their functions are distinct and complementary. For most of middle-class America, the aide function would probably be redundant. But in situations where it is needed, it appears to be both appropriate and cost-effective.[61]

Two important community programs are focused on low-income areas in Detroit and Los Angeles. In Detroit the Shared Health Education Program (SHEP), sponsored by three hospitals—Henry Ford, Metropolitan, and Detroit Osteopathic—is developing a program for a black, inner city community, Virginia Park, with a population of about twenty-thousand. Its multiple purposes include health education, consumer advocacy, and coordination of health services. SHEP's unique administrative and instructional hierarchy includes health education aides, community health agents, and multiple community inputs.[62]

In Los Angeles the King-Drew Consumer Health Education Services (CHES) has stimulated the development of multidisciplinary Preventive Health Education Teams that work through community organizations in the Watts area. Under the general direction of the Department of Community Medicine, Martin Luther King Hospital, the program is led by three health educators, including Mary Ashley, a member of this Task Force, assisted by a nutritionist and a staff of outreach workers. The program concentrates on five "modules"—maternal and infant care, accidents and homicide, high blood pressure, nutrition, and mental health. Submodules are being developed for each. The program is funded through a combination of state, county, and medical school funds.

A broader community-wide program, designed to cut across income and ethnic lines, is being planned in Pittsburgh, where the Health and Welfare Planning Association has assumed responsibility for development of an Interagency Council on Health Education and a Community Health Education and Information Center. The Vice-Chancellor, Health Professions, University of Pittsburgh, is chairman for the planning conference, an indication of the high level of professional and community support.[63]

Some university extension services are doing good jobs, especially with nutrition education. An outstanding example is Project HELP (Health Extension Learning Program) sponsored jointly by the University of Alabama in Birmingham (UAB) Medical Center, the Alabama Cooperative Extension Service of Auburn University, and the Alabama Department of Public Health. The program is run out of UAB's School of Community and Allied Health Resources. Four specially trained registered nurses, one for each Extension district in the state, direct the local programs after the local medical society and members of the medical community have met with community leaders to develop their list of priorities.[64]

In New Jersey a statewide network of hospital-based health education programs, associated with the College of Medicine and Dentistry of New Jersey, was developed under the direction of Anne Somers, Chairman of this Task Force. Each hospital funded by CMDNJ agrees to provide community, as well as patient, education programs.[65]

Iowa is another state where community, professional, and governmental influences appear to be converging to produce a series of homegrown community programs. Activities include Healthcare, a Des Moines hot line currently handling about a thousand calls a week, a multidisciplinary team of medical and osteopathic physicians and other professionals that calls itself Preventive Health Care Affiliates, and a consumer group known as Health Horizons.[66]

5.   National Health and Health-Related Agency Programs

There are today some seventy national health and health-related agencies and organizations affiliated with the National Health Council; most are doing some health education. Unlike the four categories previously discussed, these programs are not usually directed at individual patients or other consumers. Their general aim is broad public education within their respective areas of concern. In those cases where actual instructional programs are conducted, the sponsorship and instructional guidelines are usually national rather than local. The quanitity, quality, and effectiveness of these agency programs vary greatly.

Probably the best known and the most effective are the American Cancer Society, whose seven danger signals are now widely accepted, and the American Heart Association, which has succeeded in translating its nutritional concerns into a best-selling cookbook.[67] The National Foundation–March of Dimes "Family Health Record" form, distributed in many states, is a useful contribution to increasing family knowledge and responsibility.

The American Medical Association's Department of Health Education acts as an extensive resource and information center. It sponsors television and radio spots, a closed circuit television program for schools called "Inside-Out," and pamphlets on numerous topics. The Massachusetts Medical Society, among other state and local groups, is sponsoring a media "Anti-Self-Pollution" campaign.

Major contributions to health education of the public are also made by many organizations that do not usually identify themselves as health educators. The Planned Parenthood Federation of America, through the Alan Guttmacher Institute and its many state and local affiliates, has done a masterful job in the area of family planning. The National Safety Council is the acknowledged leader in accident prevention programs of all types. Its Defensive Driving Course has been taught in communities by an estimated ten thousand volunteer teachers and has probably helped contain the number of automobile accidents.[68] The name Red Cross has become synonymous with lifesaving and first aid.

Weight Watchers, Alcoholics Anonymous, and numerous less well known groups, run by the formerly obese, ex-addicts, and other reformed "sinners," have done some of the most effective work in their respective areas, sometimes succeeding where professionals have failed. The variety, vitality, and wide public support for such groups re-emphasize the difficulty of defining "consumer health education," let alone compressing it into a single discipline.

As already noted, the National Health Council, parent organization for most of the major nongovernmental agencies, is currently trying to establish the framework for a national center for health education financed in good part by, but independent of, government.[69]

6. Media Programs

Napoleon is reported to have said, "Let me write the songs of the people. I care not who writes their laws." With equal validity, it can be said that the values, mores, and health-related behavior of large segments of the American population today are influenced more by television than by our laws, schools, health or religious institutions.

According to the Surgeon General's Scientific Advisory Committee on Television and Social Behavior,

> More people watch television than make use of any other single mode of mass communication.... It would be difficult to overstate the pervasiveness of television in the U.S. Census data indicate that 96 percent of American homes have one or more television sets. The average home set is on more than six hours a day.... Frequent viewing begins at about age three and remains relatively high until about age 12. Then viewing typically begins to decline, reaching its low point during the teen years. When young people marry and have families, the time they spend viewing tends to increase and then remain stable through the middle adult years. After middle age.... it rises again.[70]

The potential of the media for consumer health education is obviously tremendous. A 1971 Harris poll, commissioned by the Blue Cross Association, found that 29 percent of the American people get most of their health and medical "information" from TV advertising, 28 percent from newspaper medical columns, 26 percent from magazines, and 25 percent from TV medical news. The media, as sources of health information, clearly exceeded physicians, who were named by only 51 percent.[71]

In a study of the impact of TV health messages (mostly commercials) on fifth and sixth grade children, Lewis and Lewis found that 70 percent were "believed," the proportion rising from 61 percent in a mostly white university experimental school to 86 percent in one where the children came from disadvantaged backgrounds. Forty-seven percent were reported as "true believers"—accepting all messages as true.[72]

Whether the net results of this impact have been primarily positive or negative is widely debated—and debatable. A 1970 survey of one commercial TV network channel in Detroit by investigators from Wayne State University School of Medicine reported that only 30 percent of the health time offered useful information, while 70 percent was inaccurate or misleading or both.[73]

In an editorial accompanying this report, the editor of the *New England Journal of Medicine* satirized TV drug ads in general:

> Because of the educational efforts of TV, we know that our wives' happiness, love, endurance, and resiliency will perpertually soar on high, provided they faithfully consume that elixir so rich in pep-infusing iron. Our own sagging spirits, too, will respond to this tonic, and each of us, aglow with ferriferous radiance, can proudly display "My wife!"
>
> In many other brief but pregnant interludes, TV sustains the nation's health. All of us, if we only heeded the counsel so unmistakably offered, could attain tranquil, dormant ecstasy; and while we sleep-sleep-sleep, we need not worry about that drip-drip-drip of stomach acid, for we know that the right little tablet will consume many times it's weight of monster gastric acid.[74]

Dr. Carter Marshall, Mt. Sinai School of Medicine and a member of this Task Force, puts the negative case much more bluntly:

> Television has a bad reputation among those interested in health education primarily because of the close ties of television to the advertising industry. Deceptive claims and misleading information are an integral part of advertising and a negative influence on health consumers and health providers alike.[75]

And Dr. and Mrs. Lewis conclude their study with these words: "If, however, 70 percent of all messages on television are not true, and 70 percent of these messages are believed by children, then television viewing, as presently programmed, might be labeled as hazardous to the health of future adults."[76]

Aside from advertising, there are two other frequent criticisms of the media, particularly of television, as related to children and health: (1) overemphasis on violence, speed, "machismo," and other forms of individual behavior that may be contributing to the self-destructive life styles discussed in Part I; and (2) inculcation of an attitude of passive acceptance totally at variance with the sense of individual responsibility that is one of the major goals of consumer health education.

On the later point, Dr. Bertrand New, a prominent child psychiatrist, has said,

> Not only psychiatrists but other physicians must be alert to the subtle but devastating messages that emanate from film and print—messages that distort, overstimulate, and promote confusing ethical values. For the child is being told: You should never suffer or struggle; if you buy the right product, your problems will be solved.
>
> To the child with a bellyache or a pile of homework, this is the wrong message. After all, a major task of human development is to learn to tolerate some degree of tension and to postpone certain gratifications while mastering new skills.[77]

Two prestigious bodies have studied the relationship between television violence and individual aggressiveness. The National Commission on the Causes and Prevention of Violence, headed by Dr. Milton Eisenhower, issued its report in 1969; the Surgeon General's Scientific Advisory Committee on Television and Social Behavior, in 1972. Neither group concluded that TV was a principal cause of the violence in modern society, but both saw it as an important contributing factor. Senator John Pastore, Chairman of the Senate Subcommittee on Communications, who initiated the Surgeon General's study, has since conducted two sets of hearings on the subject, the most recent in April 1974.[78]

Understandably, the networks are strongly opposed to any new regulation. But action, especially with respect to children's programs, is increasingly being demanded by parents and consumer groups. Pressure on the Federal Communications Commission has been mounting. Many conservatives as well as liberals who, citing the First Amendment, supported the media in opposing restrictions on pornography, are now questioning the sanctity of this defense in the case of excessive violence, at least in programming for children. A 1970, first-page story in *Variety*, spokesman for the entertainment industries, suggested that, on this issue, Archie Bunker and the liberals may line up together.[79]

For a brief discussion of the Eisenhower and Surgeon General's reports, the hearings of the Senate Subcommittee on Communications, and other studies and developments bearing on the question of violence and the health of American youth, see Appendix G.

Fortunately, TV's positive potential is now receiving more attention. The National Association of Broadcasters has begun to adopt advertising codes for children's TV and, at the 1975 annual meeting, also adopted the concept of a two-hour "family viewing time," effective September 1975, during which "gratuitous violence" and other material deemed inappropriate for children would not be shown.[80] Critics of the industry remain skeptical about implementation of these new rules and the industry's definition of inappropriate material. It is clear, however, that some remedial action is being attempted. The Task Force welcomes this development.

Television's ability to produce effective health material was demonstrated by the first-rate antismoking ads turned out during the period prior to the total ban on smoking ads. Some authorities now feel that the overall reduction in smoking would have been greater if both types of ads had been left on the air to compete for public attention.

The number of good medical documentaries has increased markedly in the last two or three years. All the networks are involved in producing these; some more than others. The Public Broadcasting System (PBS) has undertaken several major series, including "The Killers" (1973–74) and "The Thin Edge" (1975). The most widely publicized was the Children's Television Workshop series, "Feeling Good," which opened on PBS stations in November 1974. Intended to appeal to both adults and children, especially in low-income families, it tried to combine health education and entertainment.[81] Widely criticized for treating a serious subject too lightly, it closed after two months and reopened briefly with an entirely different format in April 1975.

One of the most successful TV health shows, which has been running for several years, is the Boston program, "House Call WCVB." This is a prime-time, weekly, live, hot-line show featuring a physician and patient discussing specific health problems and answering questions from the audience. It is reportedly viewed in 152,000 homes each week.[82] Dr. John Knowles, a member of this Task Force, was instrumental in launching this program and is strongly committed to the format.

A good deal of solid health information is conveyed through regular news broadcasts, feature programs such as NBC's "Not for Women Only," and even some of the theatrical shows that are produced primarily for entertainment, such as the phenomenal "Marcus Welby, M.D.," with its 35–40 million viewers.[83]

The uses of television for special purposes are virtually limitless. For example, Dr. Marshall has cabled a residence for the elderly and set up a studio in the basement of the building. From the studio the television programming is sent up to the residents of the building on a dedicated channel. The programs are planned and often produced by the residents themselves, and involvement in the planning and production of television programs has reduced the isolation of the resident population and increased their involvement in the world around them. The TV system also advises residents of health screening programs and provides health information. Videotapes of related activities are used to teach medical students and house officers better techniques for interviewing the elderly.[84]

Dr. Earl Ubell, an NBC executive and Task Force member, has repeatedly emphasized the positive potential in these various formats.

> Theatrical programs could be devised that would concentrate on well individuals with a potential for disease brought on by their current behavior. Much more could be accomplished in the public affairs, public service announcements, and commercial areas of broadcasting. The first two need additional encouragement for substantial programs and rational well-produced materials. In the areas of public service announcements, public health agencies would do well to help fund such materials.[85]

Moreover, those who are most severe in their criticism of TV impact on health are frequently those who have the greatest faith in its possible future. For example Dr. Marshall points out,

> Although much concern has been expressed over the program content of television, its greater significance lies in its technical capacity to disseminate information. It is of particular importance that television is an auditory and visual medium which makes possible for the first time the creation of a general data base shared by all segments of society, including low-income people whose normal sources of information exclude print media.[86]

Other spokesmen for the television and advertising industries have indicated their receptivity to improved health coverage. The president of the J. Walter Thompson Companies, addressing the Association of American Medical Colleges in 1974, reported the 1970 Detroit survey already mentioned, but indicated that the blame for the media's lack of achievement had to be shared by physicians and health educators.

> If, then, the potential of the mass media to deliver health information to the consumer has not been achieved, as suggested by this report [Wayne State Medical School study], due to the lack of participation of health authorities, then physicians and medical educators should regard this as a serious challenge to their public responsibility. Medical educators should join with others in the medical and scientific communities to make sure that health subjects covered by the media and the details included in such coverage are, in fact, of true medical significance and are presented in a fair, fac-

tual, and appropriate manner. At the very least we must stand as sentinels against the dissemination of inaccurate or misleading health information.[87]

Some educators who have worked with local TV stations point out, on the basis of their own experience, that if broadcast material is professionally prepared, and if skillfully approached, the stations are frequently very cooperative. Stations need to earn "Brownie points" with the Federal Communications Commission, and health education programming can often serve this function.

The Task Force would obviously prefer to see such improvement in health education programming and elimination of the negative features accomplished voluntarily. Self-regulation is always preferable to governmental regulation if it can be made effective. The evidence to date suggests that, in this area as in most others that we are concerned with, a combination of both will be needed, the ideal being self-regulation within a context of clearly defined public accountability.[88] The two parts of our Recommendation 8 are directed to this goal.

We also agree with the concluding words of the Surgeon General's Scientific Advisory Committee Report:

> The Department of Health, Education, and Welfare would do well to consider increased involvement in this field, not just in relation to the possibly harmful effects of television, but also to develop the experience and professional relationships needed to consider and stimulate television's health-promoting possiblities.[89]

HEALTH EDUCATION PERSONNEL

The wide range of consumer health education programs, summarized above, is carried on by an even wider range of professional and occupational groups and individuals engaged, on a full-time or part-time basis, in these activities. Indeed, there are some who say, "Anyone who influences health behavior is a health educator."

While this is extreme, it is equally obvious that the term "health educator" can no longer be confined to those who meet the traditional Public Health Service definition, i.e., "The practitioners of health education are public health educators and school health educators."[90] Nor is the Task Force's definition of "consumer health education" (see p. xv and Part III, p. 75) very helpful in this respect. No one individual could be expected to master all six skills or functions contained in the definition.

As a pragmatic matter, we have divided the field into two groups: (1) health education specialists—individuals who have a degree from an accredited academic program in health education, who see their role primarily as applying expertise in educational theory and methodology to health problems, and are employed full time in this type of work; and (2) all others who are engaged in carrying out one or more of the six functions set forth in our definition. The first group is, obviously, very much smaller than the second. However, they "got there first," and so we discuss them first.

Health Education Specialists

There is very little hard data on health education specialists. All figures are estimates. Even the figure for "professional" health educators given by the President's Committee on Health Education—25,000[91]—has since been disavowed.[92] However, the estimates listed below are of such an order of magnitude that they are adequate to support the conclusions.

Dr. Simonds estimates "the total number of individuals prepared in health education at the baccalaureate, masters, or doctoral levels and working actively in the field of either public health education or school health education [at] no more than 12,500 [including] no more than 2,000 prepared in community or public health education." For documentation of this estimate and a more detailed discussion of health education manpower, see Appendix F. Other estimates are even lower.

The six major professional organizations in the field report their current membership as follows:

- Society of Professional Health Educators (SOPHE)—over 1,000 community health educators;[93]
- American Public Health Association:
    Public Health Education Section—over 1,600 community health educators
    School Health Education Section—300–500 school health educators;[94]
- American Association for the Advancement of Health Education (affiliated with National Education Association)—4,000 school health educators;[95]
- American School Health Association—3,500 school health educators;[96]
- American College Health Association—180 in Health Education Section.[97]

These organizations are not mutually exclusive. Membership in two or more is common, while some educators belong to none. The figures indicate, however, the very small number of individuals who identify themselves as health educators.

A comparison of Dr. Simonds' outside estimate of 12,500 with the 1974 resident civilian population—approximately 210 million—shows one health educator per 16,800 persons. In contrast, there were, in 1973, one active physician for every 647 persons and one nurse for every 258.[98] Despite the fact that health educators are far less expensive to train than physicians and, in most cases, less expensive than nurses, clearly no national priority has been identified in this area.

Health education specialists are currently being trained at undergraduate colleges, schools of public health, and graduate schools of education. A 1974 listing identifies 124 bachelor's degree programs, 94 master's, and 31 doctor's, at a total of 139 schools.[99] The relatively large number of schools is misleading, however. In 1969–70, the last year for which information was available, the total number of master's degrees in "public" (as opposed to "school") health education granted was 160. Of these, 33 went to foreign students and 28 were from the University of Puerto Rico.[100] The number of Ph.D.'s in health education granted annually probably does not exceed two dozen.

Within the three principal degree levels, there are five major areas of concentration: (1) community health education, (2) community organization, (3) patient education, (4) school health education, and (5) health and physical education. However, as the figures indicate, the great majority of health education students end up teaching in primary and secondary schools.

It is beyond the scope of this brief report to go into questions of curriculum and other factors influencing the quality of the education currently provided to health education specialists, a subject that obviously deserves careful study. Dr. Irving Shapiro, a recognized leader of the profession and a member of this Task Force, has summarized recent developments as follows:

> Specialized training for health educators continues to expand, in schools of public health and elsewhere. It is also undergoing evaluation and change as the discipline seeks to codify the theory and knowledge unique to its efforts in a changing society.
>
> The basic behavioral sciences, psychology, anthropology, and sociology, underlie this discipline, as do to a lesser extent, the natural sciences, such as biology, physiology, and chemistry. It is the integration and application of findings from these basic sciences in the interests of better health that characterize the health educator, functioning on different levels in a variety of roles.[101]

Health education specialists (other than school health educators) are being trained primarily for planning, consultative, and academic positions rather than actual teaching or other individual consumer contacts. In the typical curriculum there is very little attention to clinical health problems or specific techniques of prevention. The emphasis is clearly on process rather than substance. Considering the small number of personnel available, this may be a sensible pragmatic adjustment. On the other hand, any profession that encourages all "chiefs" and no "Indians" runs some danger of losing its occupational base.

As to programs preparing students for school or college employment, the concluding paragraph of a recent survey of graduate programs is instructive.

> There were only two items in which there was unanimous agreement: the dissertation is required for the doctoral degree; and all doctoral programs require a written and oral examination on course work, followed by an oral defense of the dissertation. This lack of unanimity may indicate an attempt to design courses of study that will prepare the student for the type of position he desires in light of the background he brings to the program. It may also mean that either there is no established core of competencies necessary for a school/college health educator, or individuals are entering the field with such diverse backgrounds that it is difficult to show a great deal of unanimity in a study such as this.[102]

Physicians, Nurses, and Other Health Personnel

Physicians are, of course, involved in health education in many ways. Probably most of the 295,257 reported to be engaged in patient care in 1973[103] were providing some form of education to their patients. Among the various specialists, those giving more time and emphasis to health education include pediatricians, obstetricians, internists, family practitioners, psychiatrists, those engaged in rehabilitation, and general practitioners.

The Department of Family Medicine at the University of Wisconsin Medical School now includes a patient educator on the faculty and reports being involved in "research in patient education and education of residents in patient teaching at our three Model Family Practice Clinics."[104]

Physicians whose practice includes a large proportion of diabetics, patients with hypertension and heart disease, alcoholics, drug addicts, and other life-style-related conditions have been among the first to support the new emphasis on health education. Doctors in the leadership of the American Heart Association, American Cancer Society, American Diabetes Association, and a few other voluntary health agencies have done yeoman service to the public at large as well as for their own patients. As already noted, the renewed interest in primary care has also brought renewed interest in preventive medicine in general and health education in particular.

Another important group of physicians with more than a moderate interest in patient education, a group that cuts across specialty lines, are the hospital-based directors of medical education. With their dual interest in patient care and education and their experience in institutional program planning and budgeting, the directors of medical education can be invaluable allies in establishing and supervising hospital-based health education programs. In the CMDNJ New Jersey program, for example, their support has been crucial.

Physicians engaged in preventive medicine, public health, and occupational health generally have a philosophical concern with, and often even a personal commitment to, health education. The sponsorship of this Task Force by the American College of Preventive Medicine is a striking example. However, few, if any, of these doctors—most of whom operate at administrative levels—have either the time or the inclination to engage actively in educational activities, aside from an occasional lecture or seminar.

Reflecting the growing interest in life style-related illness and disability, a few psychiatrists, pediatricians, and other physicians are experimenting with new theories and techniques that have come to be called "behavior modification." Dr. Richard Bates, a member of this Task Force, has suggested that "behavioral medicine" should be the next big medical specialty.[105] If this should happen, it could mean an important new source of support for health education. At present, however, the number of patients actually reached by serious behavior modification specialists is small. For a review of recent developments in this area by Dr. Frederick Bass, a member of this Task Force, see Appendix H.

Thus, despite the impressive record of physician involvement, it is clear that we can look to the medical profession for only a small proportion of the nation's total health education needs. In the last analysis, the average physician now considers his or her primary tasks to be diagnosis and therapeutic intervention. Only when intervention fails or has limited results does he or she turn to maintenance and education. Thus, to some extent the need for education is associated with therapeutic failure, and it is not surprising that many doctors lose interest at this point.

It is hoped that medical education and professional values will gradually change to take into greater account the inevitability of widespread chronic illness and disability in a society with a rapidly falling birthrate and an ever-increasing proportion of the elderly. For the time being, however, it is obvious that the nation must look to other professions to supply most of its health education needs, even for those who are already patients.

The one profession that is now doing the most consumer health education in the United States is nursing. This is evident in the figures. There were, in 1973, 815,000 active registered nurses (there are more today), of whom 54,800 were in public health and school nursing and 20,000 in occupational health nursing.[106] Much of their work is educational.

Many, perhaps most, of the 578,000 nurses working in hospitals and nursing homes have extensive technical responsibilities and limited time to give to patient education. Nevertheless, for nurses, unlike physicians, patient education is now generally assumed to be an explicit part of the job responsibility, generally so stated in the state nursing practice acts and a component of all state licensing examinations. Moreover, the nurse, unlike the doctor, does not usually have the same professional and emotional preoccupation with diagnosis and intervention. The nurse is frequently more interested in the patient as a person and looks on maintenance and educational activities as a major challenge rather than evidence of failure.

Obviously, not all nurses feel this way. Many are following in the footsteps of the physician specialists into highly technical specialties. Others are inhibited—sometimes with good reason, often without—from giving the time or attention to patient education that they ideally would like to give. In some hospitals where nurse clinicians or others are already engaged in patient education there may be strong resentment against the introduction of a new program staffed by health educators or other "outsiders." In addition, the majority are not prepared, by either training or experience, for the administrative aspects of running a health education program.

Despite all such problems, the fact remains that owing to their numerical superiority, their general knowledge of health and illness, and their direct contact with the patient, student, or other consumer, nurses today are doing more health education than any other group. Some respected health educators maintain that this is not only a pragmatic fact but is the way it should be: most actual patient teaching should be done by nurses—under supervision of a professional "educator."[107] Another view maintains that professional nurses constitute the largest pool of potential manpower available for rapid upgrading toward expanded health education responsibilities. Graduate schools of public health already report a marked increase in the number of professional nurses in health education programs.

Among the other professional and occupational groups that are contributing in some degree to health education, the following are especially important: dentists and dental hygienists; physical, speech, and occupational therapists; pharmacists; social workers; nutritionists; and dietitians. The average dentist and dental hygienist seem more concerned with prevention and patient education than does the average physician. The dental profession as a whole has received too little credit for its consistent support of preventive and maintenance activities, including proper diet.

The 133,000 pharmacists[108] active in practice in the United States in 1973 come into frequent contact with consumers having their prescriptions filled or purchasing nonprescription drugs. Often the consumer will question the pharmacist about the impact or side effects of such drugs or may even consult him about undiagnosed symptoms. Leaders of the American Pharmaceutical Association and others have suggested that pharmacists should devote more time and attention to educating their customers,[109] and, in at least one state, New Jersey, the Medicaid program is starting to add 10 cents to the professional fee for each prescription where the pharmacist agrees to undertake such education.

The effectiveness of health education by pharmacists remains to be demonstrated. One major effort concentrated on the placement of revolving floor racks containing health information pamphlets, which were changed monthly[110] —an effort that falls far short of our definition of health education. Some students of the profession have pointed to pharmacists' errors regarding patient counseling,[111] while others have noted an improvement in patients' understanding of their illnesses and compliance with prescribed medication after such counseling.[112] In general, it is hard to conceive of any serious health education taking place in the hectic atmosphere of many modern chain drugstores. The pharmacist who wishes to engage in patient education will, almost certainly, have a better opportunity to do so if working in a hospital, HMO, or other clinical setting.

Social workers who operate in medical settings may provide health information and are often the main channel through which patient health behavior is directly approached. This is particularly true in the psychiatric field in which the social worker is an adjunct therapist directly concerned with behavior changes.

The still relatively small, but growing, number of nurse practitioners and "physicians' extenders"—physicians' assistants and associates and nurse practitioners of various types—are almost certainly doing some patient education under specific delegation from supervising physicians.

Several hundred thousand licensed practical nurses, nearly all with direct patient contacts, constitute another large pool of potential educators at the one-to-one level. So do the uncounted numbers of "outreach" workers, employed by neighborhood health centers and other community health organizations.

In the nonmedical field growing numbers of professionals are turning their attention to health behavior change. Psychologists, sociologists, and other behavioral scientists, armed with new theories and techniques of behavior modification, have increased their efforts to change life style behavior—smoking, drinking, eating—that bears heavily on health.[113] Their input is also evident in the increasingly rigorous evaluation of traditional health education techniques and in research on human behavior that leads to change modalities.

Turning to a different arena altogether, we find growing numbers of audiovisual experts and media technicians moving into the field of health education. One TV show, "Feeling Good," employed several hundred. There must be several thousand now employed by the drug and appliance manufacturers in the production and distribution of hardware and software destined for patient and community education and related screening programs.

Community activists—individuals concerned with organizing neighbor-hoods and cities for political purposes—are now more than ever focusing on health. Aside from their concern with the operation of traditional health fa-cilities, they are beginning to operate health behavior programs in drug abuse, vaccination, and other areas.

Finally, many health education programs could not survive without large numbers of volunteers. For example, as already noted, the National Safety Council's Defensive Driving Course was offered to some five million people by some ten thousand volunteer teachers.[114]

In the face of this avalanche of new personnel, it is no wonder that the two thousand or so public health education specialists often feel themselves be-leaguered and defensive—pleased by the attention suddenly being paid to a long-neglected field, but somewhat resentful of the intrusion of "outsiders." This is understandable. However, in the words of a wise physician, Dr. Roger Lee, "Medicine . . . is mobile, and many of us get breathless not so much by trying to keep up with medical progress as by trying to avoid being run over by it—the juggernaut." [115]

The rush to technological medicine of the past quarter century is now ap-parently being superseded by the rush to personalized care and behavioral change. The new juggernaut is moving, and our guess is that there will be little respect for traditional jurisdictions or credentials. The outcome of this sometimes painful confrontation—painful for both sides—is still far from clear. Will the traditional profession of health education be able to expand and develop rapidly enough to assimilate the new forces? Will the new forces overwhelm the old? Or will there be multiple approaches?

The problem goes deeper than merely a confrontation of old and new. The influx of the latter has merely dramatized the pre-existing fragmentation of the field of health education. In our classification, admittedly arbitrary, we identified six separate categories of health education programs. Others could have been added. The question is, are these subdivisions or specialty areas within a single recognized discipline, analogous to the various specialties within the profession of medicine? Or are they separate, unlinked by any common body of knowledge, let alone any common credentials?

Undoubtedly there are some commonalities among the various actors in this vast drama—the diabetologist with his patient "contract," the cardiac nurse educator, the second-grade "hygiene" teacher, the outreach worker at a neighborhood health center, the producer of "Feeling Good," and so forth. Presumably they all agree on the importance of behavioral factors in the pre-vention and management of illness and disability. Presumably they are all committed to the general proposition of "helping people to help themselves." Presumably they could all subscribe to our six-point definition of "consumer health education."

Beyond that point, however, there is clearly wide divergence—in the necessary skills, educational preparation, and credential requirements. This, of course, is equally true of the general fields of "education" and "health." Just as there is no effort today to insist on a common educational background for the kindergarten teacher and the college professor or the physician and the nurse's aide, so it would probably be equally counterproductive to insist on a single discipline of "health educator."

What we are probably witnessing is the emergence of a new "field" rather than a single new or revised "discipline." This new field represents a confluence of interests, concerns, and skills drawn not only from education and health but, very importantly, from the new consumer movement. Thus the term that we have adopted, "consumer health education" (CHE), differs in a subtle but significant fashion from older "health education"—although we continue to use the latter as a popular abbreviation.

Clarification of this issue could help greatly to clear the air for future development of the entire field. Most advocates have probably felt instinctively that CHE is too big and too complex for any one profession or occupation to claim sovereignty. But there was also concern over the lack of a single recognized discipline, a common body of knowledge. Acceptance of the concept of consumer health education as a broad "field" rather than a single "discipline" opens the way for the development of multiple professional disciplines and occupations advancing the common cause each in its own way.

Dr. Shapiro has stated this a little differently.

> Those trained as health educators, whose numbers are relatively small though growing, have long sought to encourage and assist other health workers to realize their potentials as educators.
>
> What is needed today is an organized, sustained effort to delineate effective health education programming throughout the extensive range of appropriate settings, to identify the roles that all concerned need to play, and to develop the necessary legal, academic, and financial supports. Only in this way can health education grow in a socially responsible way, improve its knowledge, skill, status, and prestige and, most profoundly, make its contribution in meeting the health needs of all the people. [116]

If this concept is accepted, the next step should be to clarify and define the major professions and occupations involved, to attempt some projections as to future needs within each, educational requirements, necessary training facilities, and funds. Clearly a major study is needed of the whole field of health education manpower. Recommendation 9 addresses this issue.

Within this general requirement, three areas appear to have special urgency:

1. development of research personnel—both M.D.'s and Ph.D's—capable of advancing behavioral sciences to the point of assuring greater effec-

tiveness in health education methodologies;

2. better and more systematic training of physicians, nurses, and other health care personnel in health education theory and methodologies; and

3. clarification of the role of the health education specialist and adjustment accordingly of the numbers being trained and the skills being acquired.

An experimental program, which addresses portions of points 2 and 3 above, is currently being developed by the CMDNJ Office of Consumer Health Education. Under a grant from the New Jersey Regional Medical Program and in cooperation with Montclair State College and a number of hospitals, a short postgraduate program to train experienced nurses and other health personnel as health education coordinators for New Jersey hospitals and other care institutions was conducted during the 1975 summer and fall terms. Officials of all four state colleges now offering health education programs have participated in developing the new curriculum, and it is anticipated that all programs will be enriched as a result.

COSTS AND FINANCING

Most health education programs are notoriously underfinanced. Personnel are generally underpaid and overworked. A statement (1971 or 1972) by the Society of Public Health Educators (SOPHE) reports average starting salaries at about $7,500, with regular salaries "around $10,000 in public agencies and a little higher in private agencies or specially funded demonstration projects." [117]

Facilities and equipment are frequently shared with other institutions and agencies. National educational campaigns have kept their costs down by using "public service" time on radio and television to carry their message. The aim—sometimes conscious, sometimes unconscious—has been to hold budgets to a level almost unnoticeable in the context of a hospital or an agency's total health expenditures.

The health education budgets of even those hospitals with organized programs are in the order of $25,000–$50,000 a year, typically about one-fourth of one percent of the institution's overall budget. An occasional institution may reach $100,000. At Monmouth Medical Center, a New Jersey hospital with one of the strongest commitments to health education in the state and firm administrative and medical staff support, the 1973 health education budget was about $34,000, or one-fifth of one percent of the overall $22 million budget. [118] The health education budget is substantially smaller than the public relations budget. This estimate does not include the unidentified cost of education provided by doctors and nurses in the normal course of patient care. But even if such expenditures could be segregated and added to the identified budget, it is doubtful if the total would amount to more than one-half of one percent.

The 1975 budget of the new Bureau of Health Education of DHEW has already been noted—$3.5 million—a little over one-tenth of one percent of the total federal health budget for this year.[119]

By way of contrast, the cost of one program—the Stanford Heart Disease Prevention Program, frequently singled out for its effectiveness—is $4 million, and the cost of a single TV series, "Feeling Good," is reported to be $7 million.[120] But even such figures pale into insignificance alongside some of the better-known advertising budgets: Alka-Seltzer—$24 million (1973); Anacin—$29 million (1974); Winston cigarettes—$22 million (1974). [121]

A few health education programs are self-supporting. Weight Watchers, for example, proved so profitable that it was recently acquired by the Pillsbury Flour Company and Smoke-Enders by the Schick Manufacturing Corporation. The cost of a Schick smoke-abatement clinic is reported to be $500. [122] Corporate enterprise apparently sees in some of these programs the opportunity for substantial profit, but the cost obviously puts them out of the reach of most smokers.

A few hospital and community programs are supported, in whole or in part, by registration fees. In some hospitals, expectant parents classes are money-makers and help to support other activities for which no fees can be charged. However, since most health education rightly slants its efforts disproportionately toward the medically deprived segments of the population, fees rarely meet the full costs.

The field of health education as a whole, despite its often absurdly low costs, faces a constant struggle for funds. Most medical care programs are refunded almost automatically because their value is taken for granted, and past budgets not only serve as precedents but are expected to increase as both quantitative growth and qualitative improvement are assumed to be desirable. But because health education programs are new—at least to the mainstream of the health care economy—they are constantly in the position of having to prove themselves and justify their existence.

What are the major sources of funding? Obviously they differ for the six categories of programs. Some are better funded and more secure than others. Occupational health programs are probably in the best position since their cost is generally passed on in the price of the product or service. By the same token, however, effective programs are all-too-often limited to large companies that are in a position to absorb or pass through the costs. Many American workers are employed in firms too small, too competitive, or otherwise unable to do so. As already noted, the Occupational Health and Safety Administration alloted $6.6 million to occupational health education programs in 1974 and 1975.

School health budgets have been expanding rapidly in recent years, and budgets for school health programs have also undoubtedly increased. The

Task Force has no hard data on this subject but, by all accounts, health education remains at the bottom of the average academic totem pole. Increased funding is badly needed, especially for research and development. The Meeds-Clark bill addresses this need with a proposed three-year authorization of $140 million; $25 million for FY 1976.

For patient education, third-party payment is clearly the method of choice. So long as such education was provided by doctors, nurses, and other health professionals as a nonidentifiable part of patient care, most third-party payers did not question reimbursement. Today, however, as more and more separate programs are established and other personnel become involved, it is harder to "bury" the educational costs, small as they are, in routine care. A move has been under way for several years to persuade all third-party payers, governmental and private, to recognize patient education as a legitimate component of patient care, one that need not hide itself but can appear as a separate item in the hospital budget or the physician's bill.

The Health Insurance Benefits Advisory Council (HIBAC) to the Secretary of HEW addressed itself to this issue in a report to the secretary, February 1974 (Appendix I). On this score, the report added nothing new but helped to clarify the position of Medicare and Medicaid. So far as Medicaid outpatients are concerned, there appears to be considerable leeway for educational activities. Not so with Medicare, or Medicaid inpatients! Any activity that has to be labelled "preventive" must be disallowed for reimbursement under existing legislation. It is still possible to "bury" such expenses and, to sweeten the picture, the Social Security Administration holds out the possibility of funding a few experimental health education projects under section 222 of P.L. 92–603. But these are, at best, emergency expediencies, not the sort of reliable funding that a sound program requires.

In August 1974 the Blue Cross Association (BCA) approved a position paper strongly endorsing the concept of patient education and urging member plans to reimburse hospitals for such activities (See Appendix J). This was a very useful document, one to be welcomed by everyone interested in health education. BCA guidelines are one thing, however, and individual plan implementation is another. Very few plans are now reimbursing for patient education as such. Of course, both Blue plans, like other carriers, do reimburse for unidentified health education provided in the normal course of physician and/or hospital care. Moreover, during the last decade, there has been a slow increase in the number of insurers willing to pay for inpatient treatment of alcoholism; and outpatient benefits, presumably including education, are clearly on the horizon.

The recession of 1974-1975 and the increasing pressure on health care providers to hold down their still rapidly rising costs have presented the health education movement with a particularly difficult problem just at the time when many third-party leaders are beginning to "turn on." The issue is now not so much bargaining between the carrier and the hospitals as intra-hospital and interprofessional bargaining.

For example, if a state imposes a ceiling on hospital Blue Cross and Medicaid reimbursement rates (an increasing number of states now have the authority to do this) or if the Social Security Administration does this for Medicare rates, there will inevitably be a struggle within the hospitals as to where the excess will be cut. In the intense competition, a new program like health education, without the firm backing of strong professional interests, is very likely to suffer. Even if the hospital administration, the medical staff, and the third-party carrier or intermediary agree on the desirability of establishing or continuing such a program, the fact that Medicare policy discourages such action—(1) by omitting patient education from the list of requirements in the official Conditions of Participation, and (2) by withholding reimbursement—is a powerful deterrent. Some way must be found to reverse this anomalous situation as well as to encourage other payers to be more aggressive in their support.

Traditionally, public and community programs were financed by grants or direct allocations from government, local united funds, voluntary agencies, or industry. This is still true of most of the new TV programs. "The Killers," "Feeling Good," "Drink, Drank, Drunk," and others have been supported by grants from the Robert Wood Johnson Foundation, Commonwealth Fund, Public Broadcasting Corporation, Exxon, the 3M Company, and others.

The President's Committee on Health Education reported that DHEW spent $30 million for "specific," and $14 million for "general," health education programs in 1973—altogether less than ¼ of 1 percent of that year's budget.[123] Some feel this understates the actual expenditures; others that the estimates are too generous. Presumably most of this money went for programs involving smoking, drug addiction, alcoholism, and related conditions.

As for philanthropic and private agency funding, Edward Van Ness, Executive Vice-President of the National Health Council, recently estimated that the voluntary health agencies spent $175–$220 million for public health education in 1973. "This does not include," he continued, "literally hundreds of millions of dollars spent by professsional associations, insurance companies and other health organizations."[124]

Let us assume that Mr. Van Ness is accurate and that professional associations, insurance companies, and others are literally spending "hundreds of millions" on health education and these should be added to his top figure for the voluntary agencies and similarly generous estimates for federal, state, and local governments. Let us assume, in short, that funds in the order of $500 million are available from these sources for public and community health education. Compared to the $118 billion we are currently spending for total health costs, expenditures on health education are still less than one-half of 1 percent of the total.

In fact, most members of the Task Force question the accuracy of these "guesstimates" and believe the total figure is closer to $250 million, which brings us back to less than one quarter of one percent—a figure consistent with the health education budgets of the more progressive hospitals.

Another problem is that most of this money is strictly earmarked. Public appeals are generally made, and funds are raised and disbursed, on the basis of categorical diseases or conditions. Local united funds have tried to get away from this overlapping and administratively wasteful approach, but with indifferent success. A community group wishing to establish a program for sickle cell screening and counseling this year may find more than enough money available for breast cancer but nothing for sickle cell. Next year, the reverse could be true. It is extremely difficult to find reliable, long-term support for any program, let alone to develop the organizational matrix or infrastructure that would permit efficient use of such funds as can be obtained.

The fact that the community hospital offers such an infrastructure and provides a ready base of operations and access to a broad spectrum of health-related resources, which do not have to be assembled from scratch each time a new program is started, is another reason that much attention is now being paid to the hospital as a major locus for community as well as patient education programs. But, even if a community program is run out of a hospital, it is probably unreasonable as well as unrealistic to expect such programs to be funded in the same way as patient education programs—through third-party payers. Of all the categories of health education, community programs are probably most desperately in need of funds.

The necessity of constant worry about where the next dollar is coming from is debilitating to administrators and to their programs. No part of the country now has the resources to develop a comprehensive network of health education programs and services. At best, a community is offered a series of small, separate programs by those institutions, agencies, and groups able to hide their programs under some other heading or to piece together a short-term grant. In addition, because existing programs have such small budgets, they frequently lack the personnel or the "clout" to defend them.

Will community health education continue to be viewed as an interesting sideshow hired week by week? Or can it achieve a secure position in the mainstream? In a field as dynamic as health, with constant changes in both supply and demand factors, as well as in the environmental context, it is obviously impossible to give any meaningful definition of "a secure position." As a practical matter, however, certain pragmatic goals and limits have to be set, both for the long-term, and the immediate future.

For the long-term, the Task Force debated the advisability of specifying a certain percentage of national health expenditures. The drawbacks to such an exercise are obvious. On the other hand, we concluded that such a target would provide a useful guide for legislative action. A range from 5–10 percent was suggested.

In the absence of a firm actuarial basis for any such figure, but believing in the symbolic value of a popular target, we agreed on a long-term goal of 6 percent, roughly one-sixteenth, of the national health budget.

Although we arrived at this figure partly through poetic license—"an ounce of prevention is worth a pound of cure"—it seems an eminently reasonable target. This means that, within a few years, we are talking about a national health education budget—public and private funds combined—in the order of $6–8 billion. If this appears unreasonable, or even shocking, it is far less so than the fact that we are already spending in the order of $118.5 billion a year for health care.[125] The hope, of course, is that the traditional ounce of prevention will help to reduce, or at least contain, the pound of cure or care.

For the immediate future, we are concerned primarily with the need for significant federal support of public and community health education, including new uses of the media, and substantial research into the still dimly understood mechanisms of behavior change.

The two general health education bills now pending in Congress (see Part I) address this major gap in national health policy in varying degrees. The Cohen-Javits bill (H.R. 3205 and S. 1521) establishes a new Health Education Administration in DHEW, reporting directly to the Secretary, and authorizes the Administrator to make grants or contracts to public or private bodies to develop or evaluate educational techniques and to develop "multifaceted systems of health care education for a defined geographic region." Authorizations are limited to $5 million for the first fiscal year, $10 million for the second, and $15 million for the third.

The Carter-Kennedy bill (H.R. 5839 and S. 1467) establishes two health education bodies: a National Center for Health Education and Promotion in DHEW and a private nonprofit Institution for Health Education and Promotion. The DHEW center would, among other duties, support research, community, and media programs and would work with Congress and other federal agencies on health education and health promotion, within an authorization limit of $35 million the first year, $40 million the second, and $45 million the third. The Institution would receive $1 million in federal funds the first year, $3 million the second, and $5 million the third.

The Task Force's own thoughts on financing are presented in Recommendation 11.

EFFECTIVENESS

There is wide disagreement as to the effectiveness of current health education efforts. The pro and con arguments are both ideological and empirical.

Some critics still cite the old bromide. "You can't change human nature!" assuming, by inference, that human beings have always driven to and from work in private cars, smoked a pack of cigarettes a day, and eaten 119 pounds of beef each year! The more sophisticated admit that individual behavior can, of course, be changed, but feel that the situation is hopeless vis-a-vis the overwhelming counterforces represented by advertising and the generally prevalent American life style. The failure of school health education to influence more positively the life style of American youth is frequently cited. Some physicians express discouragement with their efforts to help patients correct self-destructive habits.[126] Behavioral scientists disagree among themselves as to the effectiveness of different techniques of behavior change.[127]

Proponents sometimes content themselves with pointing to the shortcomings of therapeutic medicine and the increasingly obvious relationship between current health status and individual behavior. The inference is that if one approach has failed, the other must work.

More sophisticated defenders point to a growing body of literature documenting, on the basis of controlled statistical studies, the effectiveness of individual health education programs in terms of improved health status, cost savings, or both. One of the best summaries of such studies, prepared by the Blue Cross Association, concludes as follows (for full report and documentation, see Appendix J):

> With respect to health care outcomes, studies have shown the quality-increasing effects of patient education. At the University of Southern California Medical Center, the reorganization of the system of diabetic care and the initiation of a multi-faceted program of patient education was associated with a reduction of approximately two-thirds in the incidence of diabetic coma from 1968 to 1970. Similarly, in another study, a significantly higher percentage of congestive heart failure patients receiving educational support improved in their classification. Also, recent work at Massachusetts General Hospital has shown that the provision of information and guidance contributed to reduced pain among surgery patients.

With respect to costs, the Blue Cross Association reports:

> While not presenting conclusive evidence of reduced *total* costs of care for specific groups, some studies do suggest large cost savings as a result of changes in the pattern of utilization. For exam-

ple, the Tufts–New England Medical Center research, using a self-selected sample of male hemophiliac outpatients given post-period instruction and practice in self-infusion, yielded the following pre-post comparisons: Total inpatient days declined from 432 to 42, outpatient visits per patient decreased from 23.0 to 5.5, and total costs per patient went down 45 percent (from $5,780 to $3,209).

At the University of Southern California Medical Center, a reorganization of the diabetic care system, incorporating a telephone "hotline" for information, medical advice, and the filling of prescriptions, counseling by physicians and nurses, and pamphlets and posters to promote the service, was associated with more than a 50 percent reduction in emergency room visits per clinic patient and the avoidance of approximately 2,300 medication visits. These findings suggest that certain types of patient education do promote the substitution of self-care and information-seeking for acute care services.

Professor Lawrence Green, Johns Hopkins University School of Hygiene and Public Health, one of the nation's foremost exponents of health education evaluation strategies, has also reviewed the results and concludes that "the payoff is more than proportionate to the effort and costs."[128]

Data from one of the largest and most important studies yet undertaken, the Stanford Heart Disease Prevention Program sponsored by the National Heart and Lung Institute and directed by Dr. John Farquhar, of the Stanford Medical School Department of Medicine, and Dr. Nathan Maccoby, Director, Stanford Institute for Communication Research and a member of this Task Force, are just now becoming available. The objectives of this $4-million, five-year interdisciplinary study were to teach individuals between the ages of 35 and 69 about heart risk factors and to stimulate them to adopt more healthful behavior. The study is comparing risk factor decreases in three similar California communities exposed to different mixes of television spots, printed materials, and personal instruction.[129]

According to the 1974 report of the Institute for Communication Research,

> For the most part, the findings have been extremely encouraging. In general, Watsonville (the maximum-treatment town) has shown substantial change; Gilroy (the mass-media-only town) has changed a little, and Tracy (the control town) has changed negligibly or in the opposite direction. Moreover, within Watsonville, the intensively instructed respondents have changed more than have their randomized controls, who received our campaign messages only through the media and their mail boxes.[130]

Following are examples of comparative behavior changes, as reported by Drs. Farquhar and P. D. Wood, Deputy Director:
- Before the campaign only about 18 percent of the population had even a crude idea about tryglycerides. Afterward the figure was 45 percent among the Watsonville participants.
- Cigarette smoking declined about 20 percent in Watsonville, but only about 3 percent in Gilroy and was unchanged in Tracy. High-risk persons in Watsonville cut their smoking 40 percent.
- The number of eggs eaten per week declined in all three communities: 40 percent in Watsonville, 27 percent in Gilroy, and 17 percent in Tracy. The latter figure suggests that factors other than the campaign, such as inflation, were involved.

These results led Drs. Farquhar and Wood to conclude that an educational campaign directed at an entire community can produce "striking increases in the level of knowledge of heart disease and risk factors and very worthwhile improvements in risk factor levels."[131]

This *is* encouraging, both in terms of the outcome and our ability to measure outcomes. Moreover, some respected authorities are now saying that we have overestimated the obstacles and underestimated actual achievements. For example, Dr. Carter Marshall, a member of this Task Force, concludes, on the basis of a two-year study of health education and mass communications, "Health education efforts using television rarely seem to meet the extraordinarily high expectations of health professionals, yet most do far better than even the most heavily-backed advertising campaign."[132]

As to the inherent difficulties of evaluating health education programs, Dr. Richard Podell, a member of the Task Force, has written:

> On epidemiological grounds it is clear that the evaluation of health education intervention is not fundamentally different from the evaluation of other clinical therapies. Often, it is difficult to set up the controls. However, there are many cases in which a rigorous controlled study is fairly straightforward conceptually. The only difficulty is that the investigator must have the will and the resources to create a valid study. Hundreds of such studies are performed in the evaluation of pharmacotherapy each year. The problems of randomization, long term follow-up, dropping out, subjective responses, double blinding, are almost identical. The problem is not so much that health education cannot be evaluated rigorously, but that very few have had the interest and resources to do it. The logistics, I cannot overstress, are not more formidable than those in other well controlled epidemiological studies.[133]

Perhaps the most persuasive judgment on the whole question of effectiveness comes from the Kaiser Foundation Medical Care Program. As already noted, this prototype HMO, with its 2.5 million members and $632,000,000 budget (1974), has been conducting limited health education activities, as part of a general program of prevention, for nearly three decades. Apparently Kaiser feels that the effort not only has been worthwhile but should be expanded. Its 1974 annual report, devoted entirely to "Preventive Medicine," concludes:

> Doctors in each of the six regions of the Kaiser-Permanente Program are attempting to improve or broaden the preventive services currently made available to members: namely, immunizations to control communicable diseases and early detection and intervention for chronic illnesses . . . .
> Another area of great promise is health education . . . . The program is continuing to develop educational programs designed to help the individual learn about his body and about the things that influence his health . . . . Working with public and voluntary agencies, Permanente physicians promote community-wide education programs to motivate people to develop improved life styles and to seek medical attention at the first warning signal.[134]

The chief significance of this cautiously optimistic statement is that it reflects a dollars-and-cents judgment. Kaiser educational programs have not been supported by public or philanthropic grants or subsidies. They are paid for entirely out of members' dues and are subject to the harsh judgment of the annual balance sheet.

Despite all this encouragement, it is our feeling that the significance of the few definitive studies of the effectiveness of current techniques of education and behavior change—probably no more than twenty-five to fifty altogether—should not be overstated. Nor should the difficulties of definitive measurement be underestimated; nor the strength of the countervailing forces. Despite the antismoking campaigns, the percent of teenage boys (12-18) smoking rose from 14.7 percent in 1968 to 15.8 percent in 1974. For girls the same age, the rise was from 8.4 percent to 15.3 percent.[135] Despite the widespread availability of screening programs for breast and cervical cancer, only half of American women over 17 had such tests in 1973 and nearly one-fourth had never had a breast examination.[136] The proportion of individuals taking advantage of any such screening is reported to be leveling off at about three-fourths.[137] Immunization rates also seem to have reached a peak, and some, such as polio, have dropped significantly.[138] The relationship between these figures and the lack of firm professional consensus on screening and immunization is discussed below.

As already noted, the recent decline in heart disease is attributed by leading cardiologists to public education campaigns by the American Heart Association and others. But this is virtually impossible to prove statistically. In short, we do not know, *for sure*, whether the record would have been better, or worse, or no different, if there had been no educational effort. Would there be even more smokers today if there had been no campaign? More drug abusers if no drug education? More hypertension if no screening programs? More heart attacks if the American Heart Association had not been so vigilant?

Health educators, under the leadership of Dr. Green, Dr. Podell, and others have tried to respond to this challenge positively. Determined efforts have been made to design and implement precise methodologies for measuring the impact of a given program in terms of the health status of participants and the costs. For a summary of current evaluation techniques and problems, see Appendix L. This effort to improve the state of the art of health education evaluation should be pursued with as much discipline and rigor as possible and with far more adequate financial support than in the past.

Despite these efforts, however, the Task Force is forced to conclude that, in many situations, it is as difficult to quantify and measure the outcome of health education as it is to quantify and measure the outcome of health care. Health, like life, is too complex to lend itself easily to precise measurements. Health education is far more complex than pharmacotherapy. The number of variables impinging on individual motivation,[139] behavior, and health will probably continue to defy fine statistical discrimination.

Moreover, there are dangers inherent in overemphasis on quantitative evaluation. There is already some tendency on the part of funding agencies and others to emphasize programs that lend themselves to quantitative measurement rather than those that are more broadly significant.

The chairman of this Task Force has stated elsewhere:

> We must be prepared to subject ourselves to meaningful evaluation and to accept the consequences even when the studies tell us that our programs have not met their goals. However, we cannot be so lacking in the courage of our convictions that we allow ourselves to be scared out of experimentation or subjected to more rigorous evaluation than other elements of the health care system . . . . We will never move toward a more sensible balance between preventive and therapeutic medicine if those who believe in the former commit statistical harakiri.[140]

There is even some danger that overemphasis on statistical evaluation can lead to inadequate attention to "common sense" evaluation as an ongoing managerial tool. In a provocative study that attempts "to evaluate evaluations," Professor B. A. Rocheleau concludes that much of the present effort in a related field, community mental health centers, has been wasted. The results are rarely used, he says, to influence budgetary or personnel decisions, are done primarily to pacify funding agencies, and "have had strikingly little substantive effect on the operations of these organizations."[141]

This should not be interpreted as a downgrading of evaluation efforts. On the contrary, the Task Force believes they should be strongly encouraged. We do say, however, that outcome evaluation is only one of many tools available for appraisal of policies and programs on the part of those responsible— individual program managers, bureau chiefs, Congressmen, and others.

In conclusion, it appears that two generalizations with respect to effectiveness are justified. First, consumer health education can point to a number of carefully documented success stories that can be interpreted as having reasonably wide application to similar programs. These primarily involve individuals who already have some strong motivation: patients with a chronic illness or disability, those facing an acute crisis such as surgery or childbirth, or employees whose livelihood may depend on overcoming alcoholism or some other job-threatening condition. The effectiveness of programs directed to the general asymptomatic public is far more difficult to measure, although even the modest gains with respect to cigarette smoking, coronary disease, and cancer are encouraging. So, too, is the growing volume of serious research with respect to behavior change and the increasing emphasis on evaluation.

Second, if individual behavior change programs are to be generally effective, they must be accompanied by national policies and mass communication programs designed to reinforce, rather that undermine, the message of health education. The results of the Stanford Program are particularly important in demonstrating the need for mutual reinforcement between individual and mass communications efforts.

EXTERNAL PROBLEMS

Decisions involving health education program development, methodologies, manpower, research, funding, and evaluation cannot be made in a vacuum, only by health educators and others identified with the field. The frequently inhospitable physical and cultural environment, the overwhelming national commitment to cure rather than prevention, the continuing emphasis on professional intervention rather than consumer responsibility, the widespread lack of confidence in health education, and other external obstacles are all important contributing factors to its current weakness. Internal reforms will inevitably depend, in good part, on changes in the external environment that will determine the constraints within which the internal decisions have to be made.

The same point was strongly emphasized by the Task Force on Consumer Health Behavior, a subcommittee of the President's Committee on Health Education.

> This report has repeatedly stressed the futility of relying on consumer education as performed through special educational programs for producing extensive changes in consumers' health behavior since such changes can be expected to occur only if supported and reinforced by other sources of communication and by experiences with the health care and other systems that are compatible with the educational thrust. Any discrepancies among the various sources of communication or any conflicts between educational input and actual experiences create doubts, confusion, and resistance concerning these educational efforts.[142]

To emphasize the importance of external factors, it may be useful to summarize several major external obstacles.

1. *The persistence of poverty, racial discrimination, slum housing, urban squalor, serious crime, and other health-threatening conditions largely beyond the power of the individual to control.* Considerable emphasis was placed, in Part I, on the health-threatening aspects of affluence and the rapid rise in discretionary income that characterized most of the past two decades. Along with the dramatic rise in national and family income, however, there has persisted a substantial amount of poverty with all its attendant ills. Millions of Americans, especially blacks, Puerto Ricans, Chicanos, Indians, and other minorities, have continued to remain at higher-than-average risk for infectious diseases, nutritional deficiencies, high infant mortality, and other conditions historically associated with poverty.[143] The persistent serious unemployment, along with simultaneous inflation, threatens additional millions with at least temporary poverty.

Efforts at individual health education and behavior change in the squalid ghettos of Harlem, South Chicago, Newark, South Bronx, Brooklyn, and other urban centers cannot be expected to succeed without accompanying major changes in the external environment. Does the definition of health education include advocacy of such change? The Task Force believes strongly that it does.

2. *The prevalent mores of affluent, self-indulgent, frequently violent American society.* The social milieu in which an individual finds himself has

a powerful influence on what he eats, what drugs he takes, how much exercise or physical activity he can get, how he expresses aggressive feelings—in short, on his health behavior. Despite current economic woes, the dominant cultural theme in America still emphasizes an affluent, self-indulgent, sedentary but frequently violent life style. For a background statement regarding the effects of violence on the health of American youth, see Appendix G.

Any health education program that challenges these dominant attitudes, for example, that attempts to promote safety devices in automobiles, to reduce beef consumption, and to promote gun controls faces great difficulties and often heavy opposition from both producers and consumers. Middle-class school children and teenagers often appear almost as trapped, in terms of health-threatening behavior, as the children of the ghetto. Older people, regardless of income, have difficulty finding adequate sources of healthy recreation. For tens of thousands of widows and other single women an evening walk in a city street or park has become an intolerable danger rather than a source of much-needed exercise.

Various subcultures also influence life styles that have strong antihealth components. Examples abound: high alcohol intake among the Irish; high caloric intake among Jews; among Latins, "machismo" attitudes that increase risk-taking. Paradoxically, even the remnants of Puritanism can interfere with realistic health behavior change. Veneral disease prevention, for example, is inhibited in many parts of the country because the only acceptable preventive technique that can be advocated is abstinence.

These are areas where reformers should tred with extreme caution. The rights to privacy and to ethnic cultural diversity and those guaranteed in the First Amendment and other cherished articles in the Bill of Rights are involved. But there are other, less defensible, factors as well. We are reluctantly forced to agree with a recent editorialist who wrote,

> Scientific scepticism is most frequently aimed at those whose ideas are not backed by multi-million dollar advertising budgets. Let one mother demand that the schools serve whole wheat bread and a thousand sceptical academics will take the microphone to claim that whole wheat bread has not been proved superior to white bread. But when ITT-Continental backs Wonder bread with two million dollars worth of advertising, scientists rarely demand evidence from ITT that our children should be eating white bread.[144]

The issue with which we are concerned, however, is not money, or advertising budgets, or free enterprise economics. We are concerned with the health of the American people and what we can do, through health education, to alter their behavior patterns in such a way as to protect and improve their health. To this end we cannot close our eyes to the impact of irresponsible advertising and overemphasis on violence, especially in programs designed for children.

Any effort to mount an effective consumer health education program in the United States will have to concern itself not only with individual behavior but with the social milieu and the prevalent mores that contribute to such behavior. In the words of Dr. Ubell, "Any behavior change program must include efforts to arrange the mechanical or environmental situation so that individuals who are led to change their behavior can actually do so."[145]

3. *The lack of professional consensus on major health issues.* The population as a whole is exposed to a great deal of conflicting information and has no clear idea whom to believe. Part of the confusion results from advertisers who get away with saying, for example, that one brand of aspirin is superior to another, but a large part of it stems from unresolved issues in the medical community itself.

Almost every major public health education effort by one group of physicians is accompanied by a chorus of dissent from others. The difference of professional opinion on the "cholesterol hypothesis" is well known and provides a ready excuse for consumers who are reluctant to cut down on steak and eggs. The disagreements on the value of regular exercise, annual physical examinations, periodic screening, and even some immunizations provide justification for those who prefer to put off such preventive measures. Differences of opinion on vitamins, sweeteners, and certain food additives are widely reported.

Even in the area of diabetes education, where physician leadership has been outstanding, many patients are confronted with agonizing uncertainties. Pills currently being prescribed for more than 1.5 million Americans have recently been labeled hazardous and capable of causing premature death from heart disease.[146] An editorial in the *Journal of the American Medical Association* estimates the possible number of such deaths at 10,000–15,000 a year.[147] A few weeks after the appearance of this editorial, the president of the Southern California Branch of the American Diabetes Association was reported to have said in an interview, "One-third of the patients I see who have been diagnosed as diabetic are not diabetic and never have been."[148]

In a field as dynamic as modern medicine, uncertainty and changing theories are inevitable and often a sign of new knowledge. They cannot and should not be suppressed. No sensible consumer or health educator would ask this. At the same time it must be recognized that, under present conditions, both consumer and educator are frequently being asked to accept, virtually on faith, the alleged omniscience of the physician, an omniscience that, as we have just seen, is not always justified. Perhaps this is one reason for the continued ambivalence of the medical profession with respect to consumer health education.

The remedy for this situation, in our view, is not less education and responsibility for the consumer/patient but more; not less education and responsibility for the educator but more.[149]

The educator is clearly being asked, at least implicitly, to assume responsibility for the effectiveness of the basic preventive and treatment modalities to which the educational programs are related as well as his own educational theories and techniques. Since this is so, educators should welcome current PSRO programs and other efforts to assess and control the quality of medical care. As Dr. Podell puts it,

> Any assessment of the effectiveness of health education should be prefaced by assessment of the recommendations and practices of health scientists and physicians as to what constitutes behavior which promotes health. This is essential because these recommendations and practices usually determine the substantive goals of health education programs . . . . The commitment to adequate evaluation at the level of behavior change is inextricably linked to adequate evaluation at the level of health status results.[150]

4. *The absence of organized consumer support.* The growing demand on the part of individual consumers for more and better health information and education was noted in Part I. For the most part, this demand has been directed at individual physicians, nurses, and other members of the traditional health care team or at the media. There has been a conspicuous lack of consumer interest in anything specifically called "health education." Organized labor, senior citizens, and other consumer groups that have long worked for more and better health insurance, HMOs, and other efforts to improve access to health care have not only shown little interest in health education but have, on occasion, indicated suspicion of the would-be educators.

The reasons for this apparent paradox are complex. They relate partly to the general public overemphasis on therapeutic medicine; partly to the fact that it is much easier politically to criticize doctors and hospitals for the shortcomings in our national health than to assign the major blame to consumers themselves; partly to a vague suspicion that health educators and behavioral scientists want to "take all the fun out of life" and impose some new form of Puritanism; and partly to the fact that health educators have not, until very recently, concerned themselves with the underlying environmental and socioeconomic factors that still contribute so greatly to U.S. health problems, especially of low-income groups.

We have tried, in this report, to address all of these factors in one way or another. There remains, however, one important issue that has been implied throughout but now needs to be stated explicitly: the relationship of consumer health education to consumer participation on health care policy boards and advisory committees.

In our view, the two are inextricably linked. The ultimate aim of both is the development of a well-informed, responsible, effective consumer. In the one case, the objective is better individual health; in the other, better health care institutions. Success in either of these objectives is difficult without simultaneous progress in the other. No consumer can be truly effective on a hospital or Blue Cross board unless he knows something about the processes of health and disease and what care institutions can, and cannot, be expected to accomplish. The surest way for any individual to acquire such knowledge is through personal experience. Conversely, no individual patient or other consumer can be expected to assume effective responsibility for his own health unless he feels some positive relationship to the care institutions on which he depends for guidance and in emergencies. In the past, this interrelationship has too often been neglected.

Drs. Breslow and Miller prefaced the conclusion to their 1972 American Public Health Association Inquiry into Health Services for Americans with a quotation from John Dewey.

> No matter how ignorant any person is, there is one thing he knows better than anybody else, and that is where the shoes pinch his own feet, and that is because he is the individual that knows his own troubles, even if he is not literate or sophisticated in other respects. The idea of democracy as opposed to any conception of aristocracy is that every individual must be consulted in such a way, actively or passively, that he himself becomes a part of the process of authority, of the process of social control; that his needs and wants have a chance to be registered where they count in determining social policy.

Among the conclusions that followed:

> Consumers have no real or effective role in the planning, organization, or delivery of health care . . . .
> Consumers have few meaningful options in health care today . . . .
> Consumers must be able to establish goals, objectives, and priorities of the newly-structured delivery system and make them effective in the organization and delivery of health services.[151]

The Task Force agrees and believes that health education has an important role to play in this respect. We believe that "consumerism," for all its shortcomings, can be a positive force for good health and health-related behavior.[152] We have deliberately emphasized the term in our title and in our definition of consumer health education.

5. *National policies conflicting with the goals of health and health education.* Examples have been cited throughout this report. Probably the most conspicuous is the extreme imbalance between the proportion of national health resources devoted to prevention and that devoted to cure. Other areas marked by such anomalies include national food and nutrition policies, housing, communications, control of violence, tobacco subsidies, and product advertising. If consumer health education is to have a chance of success, it must broaden its scope to include advocacy of national policies that are consistent with the goals of health and health education.

Advocacy of specific health promotion policies is beyond the charge or resources of this Task Force. Individual members have submitted proposals or statements dealing with violence (Appendix G), atherosclerotic heart disease (Appendix M), hypertension (Appendix N), nutrition education (Appendix O), and financial incentives (Appendix P), which we believe deserve serious attention. We commend these statements to the attention of the National Conference on Preventive Medicine, Congress, the Administration, and others concerned with the health of the American people. We also commend two statements indicating the potentially creative relations between consumer health education and public health regulation: one by Dr. Milton Terris, Chairman, Department of Community and Preventive Medicine, New York Medical College,[153] the other by Dr. Alexander Schmidt, Commissioner, Food and Drug Administration.[154]

NEED FOR NATIONAL LEADERSHIP

Even more important than advocacy of any particular reform or health promotion policy is the development of effective leadership and "centers of responsibility" for the ongoing study and development of such policies as well as guidance and assistance for the entire field of health education. For example, on the basis of current knowledge derived from insurance experience, epidemiological and experimental studies, it should now be possible to set specific national priority goals for 1980, 1985, and on into the future, with respect to behavior change and improvement in the incidence of most of the major chronic illnesses.

In the words of Dr. Fred Bass, a member of this Task Force,

> Setting such goals on first consideration might seem to require
> an authoritarian or even totalitarian regime. On the contrary, after

assessing the following: (1) the proportion of the population who, given full information pro and con, wish to change a particular habit or life style factor, (2) the efficacy of services designed to help those who wish to change a particular life style, and (3) the availability of personnel and facilities to provide such services, people can reasonably and democratically decide upon future, achievable target levels of those behaviors that are undesired. This and other nations have changed social behavior with respect to slavery, child labor, unhealthy housing, sewage, abject poverty, child abuse, hookworm (wearing shoes), goiter (iodine consumption), and tuberculosis (spitting). It would seem that we can achieve similar results with now-prevalent unhealthful behaviors.

Setting such goals is a task for the highest form of politics—policy-formation by consumers, by their elected representatives, by health professionals, and by those whose occupation (e.g. tobacco growers) is at stake.[155]

In theory, the entire health division of DHEW—the Public Health Service—under the Assistant Secretary for Health, is devoted to health promotion. See statement of organization and functions of the assistant secretary, Appendix Q; and the DHEW organization chart, Appendix R. In practice, however, less than 2 percent of the estimated 1975 federal health budget was devoted to prevention or disease control (Appendix B). What is true of the budget is also true of the Department's human resources.

The need for one or more such "centers of responsibility" has been recommended by students of health care and health education for years[156] and is now widely recognized. Four approaches have emerged during the past year: (1) the establishment of the Bureau of Health Education (BHE) in the Center for Disease Control (CDC), (2) the National Health Council's proposal for a single private-sector National Center for Health Education,[157] (3) the Cohen-Javits bill's proposal for a Health Education Administration that, like the present BHE, would be in DHEW but at a much higher level; and (4) the Carter-Kennedy bill's double-barrel proposal for a high-level National Office for Health Education and Promotion in DHEW along with a private but publicly-funded Center for Health Education and Promotion. Of these four approaches, we find that the Carter-Kennedy bill comes closest to meeting the requirements as we see them.

The CDC Bureau of Health Education is an anomaly. The official statement of mission and functions is broad and comprehensive (Appendix S). However, its subordinate location within the HEW hierarchy and its minuscule budget—$3.5 million in FY 1975—contradict the broad mandate and force us to question the seriousness of the present commitment. Moreover, its constituency is too narrow, largely confined to traditional public health educators.

The National Health Council's proposal deserves careful consideration as one approach to a private-sector center. However, it does not address itself at all to the need for an expanded federal effort.

The Cohen-Javits bill served an extremely useful purpose—breaking, for the first time, the Congressional ice for serious health education legislation. However, comparison of its provisions with those of the Carter-Kennedy bill indicates that the latter comes much closer to our own recommendations. Note, for example, the emphasis on health promotion as well as health education; the broader and more carefully delineated functions assigned to the proposed HEW center; the legislative base for a private-sector center; the emphasis on research; the requirement of patient education in all federally funded health care institutions; the special attention to the communications media; the proposed Interdepartmental Committee on Health Education and Promotion; and the far more adequate funding.

On the other hand, there is at least one provision of the Cohen-Javits bill that meets one of our recommendations in a way that the Carter-Kennedy bill does not: the provision for grants to develop "multifaceted systems of health care education for defined geographic regions." Both bills propose statuatory advisory councils; the Carter-Kennedy approach seems more workable. While the funds proposed in this bill are still not adequate, they are at least far more so than any alternative proposal currently being considered. For analysis of the Carter-Kennedy bill by Congressman Carter, see Appendix T.

We are not now endorsing this bill or any other specific legislative proposal. Among other reasons, it was introduced too late to permit a careful study by the entire Task Force. There are aspects of H.R. 5839 and S. 1467 that we feel should be improved, including the nomenclature and some of the provisions relating to the private sector center. We are very pleased, however, at its introduction and look forward to continued hearings thereon.

Meanwhile, we also believe there are specific functions related to consumer health education that should be assigned to CDC as well as the National Center for Health Statistics. Both agencies have important roles to play in the continuing development of a federal CHE capability.

Notes

1. E. Kasey and E. McMahon, "Education as a Living Process," in American Hospital Association, *Health Education in the Hospital* (Chicago: American Hospital Association, 1965), p. 9.

2. American Hospital Association, *Statement on the Role and Responsibilities of Hospitals and Other Health Care Institutions in Personal and Community Health Education* (Chicago: American Hospital Association, 1974).

3. National Education Association and American Medical Association, Joint Committee on Health Problems in Education, *Health Education: A Guide for Teachers and a Text for Teacher Education* (Washington, D.C., 1961), p. 7.

4. President's Committee on Health Education, *Report*, Department of Health, Education, and Welfare, 1973, p. 17.

5. S. K. Simonds, Dr. P.H., "Health Education in the Mid-70's—State of the Art," paper prepared for Task Force IV, December 1974. See Appendix C.

6. College of Medicine and Dentistry of New Jersey, Office of Consumer Health Education, "The CMDNJ-OCHE Program in Consumer Health Education," January 1975.

7. Charles Edwards, M.D., "Statement," in *Federal Focus on Health Education: Conference Proceedings*, Department of Health, Education, and Welfare, Center for Disease Control, June 1974, p. 6.

8. U.S., Office of Management and Budget, *The Budget of the United States Government, Fiscal Year 1975* (Washington, D.C.: Government Printing Office, appendix, p. 392).

9. Horace Ogden, testimony before Task Force on Consumer Health Education, Chicago, November 13, 1974.

10. *Budget of the United States Government, FY 1975,* p. 119.

11. Ibid., appendix, p. 395.

12. Ibid., p. 140.

13. Casper W. Weinberger, "The Role of the Federal Government in Educating the Public about Health," *Journal of Medical Education*, February 1975, pp. 138–42.

14. *Budget of the United States Government, FY 1975,* appendix, p. 142.

15. Russell Levering, U.S. Department of Agriculture, Agricultural Stabilization and Conservation Service, Tobacco Division, Washington, D.C., telephone communication, January 3, 1975.

16. S. K. Simonds, "Health Education As Social Policy," *Health Education Monographs*, (San Francisco: Society of Public Health Educators) vol. 2, supp. 1, 1974, pp. 1–10.

17. W. W. Marsh, M.D. and L. V. Perlman, M.D., "Understanding Congestive Heart Failure and Self-Administration of Digoxin," abstracted in A. I. Wertheimer and M. C. Smith, *Pharmacy Practice: Social and Behavioral Aspects* (Baltimore: University Park Press, 1974), p. 202.

18. T. F. Williams, M.D., "Needs for Diabetes Education," chap. 1 of G. Steiner, M.D. and P. Lawrence, "Handbook on the Education of the Diabetic Patient" (forthcoming).

19. D. L. Sackett, M.D., chairman, "A Workshop Symposium: Compliance with Therapeutic Regimens," McMaster University Medical Center, Hamilton, Ontario, May 1974 (processed), p. 3. This volume includes an extensive annotated bibliography.

20. Marsh and Perlman, "Understanding Congestive Heart Failure," pp. 202–03.

21. E.g., American Hospital Association, George Reader, M.D., conference chairman, *Strategies for Patient Education*, 2d Invitational Conference, Chicago, October 1969 (Chicago: American Hospital Association).

22. I. S. Shapiro, Ph.D., "HMOs and Health Education," *American Journal of Public Health*, vol. 65, May 1975, pp. 469–73.

23. P.L. 93–222, sect. 1301 (c) (9).

24. E.g., C. S. MacColl and C. H. Smith, *Health Education in the Health Maintenance Organization*, monograph prepared for Department of Health, Education, and Welfare, Group Health Cooperative of Puget Sound, Seattle, Washington, May 1974 (processed).

25. M. L. Schropp, "Patient Education," *Group Practice*, September-October 1974.

26. L. C. Robbins, M.D. and J. H. Hall, M.D., *How to Practice Prospective Medicine* (Indianapolis: Methodist Hospital of Indiana, 1970).

27. D. D. Etzwiler, M.D., ed., *Education and Management of the Patient with Diabetes Mellitus* (Elkhart, Indiana: Ames Co., 1973). Samples of the "contract" are available from the same source as "Guidelines for the Diabetes Health-Care Team."

28. K. W. Sehnert, M.D. and M. Osterweis, "A Concept for Health Education," *Continuing Education,* October 1974; K. W. Sehnert and J. T. Nocerino, "Course Guide for the Activated Patient," Georgetown University School of Medicine, Washington, D.C.

29. A. J. Stunkard, M.D., "New Treatments for Obesity: Behavior Modification," in G. A. Bray, M.D. and J. E. Bethune, M.D. eds., *Treatment and Management of Obesity* (New York: Harper & Row, 1974), pp. 103–16.

30. D. H. Kucha, *Guidelines for Implementing an Ambulatory Consumer Health Information System: A Handbook for Health Education* (Ft. Sam Houston, Texas: U.S. Army–Baylor University Program in Health Care Administration, 1973).

31. American Public Health Association, Resolutions and Position Papers, "Education for Health in the School Community Setting," *American Journal of Public Health,* vol. 65, February 1975, p. 201.

32. S. Blumenthal, M.D. and M. J. Jesse, M.D., "Prevention of Atherosclerosis: A Pediatric Problem," *Hospital Practice,* April 1973, pp. 81–90.

33. Arthur Krosnick, M.D., "Dispensing Medications in School," editorial, *Journal of the Medical Society of New Jersey,* vol. 71, September 1974, p. 635.

34. President's Committee on Health Education, Report, p. 21; Simonds, "Health Education As Social Policy," pp. 6–7; City of New York, Health Services Administration, Comprehensive Health Planning Agency, "Summary of Findings and Recommendations of the CHPA Study of Health Services in N.Y.C. High Schools," November 1974.

35. Steven Jerritt, Director, American School Health Association, Kent, Ohio, telephone communication, January 3, 1975.

36. Jon Fielding, M.D., M.P.H., *Economically and Culturally Targeted Health Education for Adolescents,* Department of Health, Education, and Welfare, Health Services Administration, Bureau of Quality Assurance, October 1974 (processed); U.S., Department of Labor, Manpower Administration, *Job Corps: Health Education Program Coordinators' Handbook,* Washington, D.C.

37. C. L. Marshall, M.D. and A. M. Lewis, Jr., "The Student Health Opportunities Program at the Mount Sinai School of Medicine," *Health Services Reports,* March-April 1974, pp. 152–61; C. L. Marshall, "Minority Students for Medicine and the Hazards of High School," *Journal of Medical Education,* vol. 48, February 1973, pp. 134–40; C. L. Marshall, S. Margolis, and A. M. Lewis, "Curriculum Outline for Secondary Education Through Health Program 1974–75" (processed).

38. C. E. Lewis, M.D. and M. A. Lewis, "Impact of Television Commercials on Health-Related Beliefs and Behaviors of Children," *Pediatrics,* vol. 53, March 1974, pp. 431–35, C. E. Lewis and M. A. Lewis, "Kids vs. Commercials," *Family Physician* (forthcoming).

39. C. E. Lewis, M.D., telephone communication, April 11, 1975.

40. See Simonds, Appendix F.

41. W. C. Sutton, "Status of State Certification in Health Education," appendix C in Donald A. Read and Walter H. Greene, *Creative Teaching in Health* (New York: Macmillan Co., 1971), pp. 420–28.

42. R. L. Davis, "Innovations in School Health Education in the U.S.A.," paper presented at the Eighth International Conference on Health Education, International Union for Health Education, Paris, France, July 8, 1973.

43. Robert Hendrickson, "That Healthy Summer of 1974," *Prism*, July 1975, pp. 26–32.

44. Terry Sanford, Governor of North Carolina, "Educating the Public about Health: The Role of Formal Education," *Journal of Medical Education*, January 1975, pp. 3–10.

45. E.g., E. C. Pierson, M.D., *Sex Is Never an Emergency: A Candid Guide for College Students* (Philadelphia: University of Pennsylvania, 1970); H. Z. Bennett, ed., *The Well Body Student Health Manual*, produced by students and Student Health Service Staff of the University of California, Berkeley (Berkeley: University of California, 1974).

46. For historical perspective, see, H. M. Somers and A. R. Somers, *Workmen's Compensation: The Prevention, Insurance, and Rehabilitation of Occupational Disability* (New York: Wiley, 1954).

47. J. A. Schoenberger, M.D., "How Industry Can Cut Costs of Employee Heart Attacks," *Commerce*, June 1968.

48. Sidney Wolfe, M.D., Director, Health Research Group, testimony before Task Force on Consumer Health Education, Chicago, November 13, 1974.

49. Marilyn Powers, U.S. Department of Labor, Occupational Safety and Health Administration, Office of Training and Education, Washington, D.C., telephone communication, December 13, 1974.

50. U.S., Department of Labor, Occupational Safety and Health Administration, Office of Training and Education, *Training Contracts for FY 1975* (processed).

51. Allan Kaplin, United Mine Workers Information Service, Washington, D.C., telephone communication, January 3, 1975.

52. Richard E. Nicholson, Director, Guy Phelps Health Center, Connecticut Mutual Life Insurance Company, Hartford, Connecticut, telephone communication, January 3, 1975.

53. Paul McGuire, Alcohol and Drug Rehabilitation Program Administrators, Scoville Manufacturing Company, Waterbury, Connecticut, telephone communication, January 3, 1975.

54. Commission on Chronic Illness, 1951, cited in *Preventive Medicine*, June 1973, pp. 187, 188.

55. *Ibid.*, p. 181.

56. L. G. Dales, G. D. Friedman, and M. F. Collen, "Evaluation of a Periodic Multiphasic Health Checkup," *Methods of Information in Medicine*, vol. 13, July 1974, p. 145.

57. Schoenberger, "How Industry Can Cut Costs of Employee Heart Attacks."

58. National Academy of Sciences—National Research Council, Committee for the Study of Inborn Errors of Metabolism, "Genetic Screening: Programs, Principles, and Research" (forthcoming); National Academy of Sciences—National Research Council, Committee for the Study of Inborn Errors of Metabolism, *Genetic Screening: Procedural Guidance and Recommendations* (Washington, D.C.: National Academy of Sciences, 1975).

59. A. R. Somers, N. Bryant, W. Stender, W. Frist, "Can a Hot Line Get Too Hot? " letter to the *New England Journal of Medicine*, April 11, 1974, pp. 863–64.

60. E. J. Salber, M.D., Department of Community Health Sciences, Duke University Medical Center, "Community Health Facilitator Report," Durham, N.C., 1975 (processed), p. 1.

61. R. E. Knittel, C. C. Child, and J. Hobgood, "Role and Training of Health Education Aides," *American Journal of Public Health*, vol. 61, August 1971, pp. 1571–80; W. Hoff, "Resolving the Health Manpower Crisis—A Systems Approach to Utilizing Personnel," paper presented to the annual meeting of the American Public Health Association, Institute for Health Research, October 1970.

62. Harry Dalsey, Coordinator, SHEP, "A Unique Trio Supports the Development of Community Health Education Program," paper presented to the annual meeting of the American Public Health Association, October 1974 (processed).

63. Health and Welfare Planning Association, Pittsburgh, *Newsletter*, December 1974.

64. University of Alabama in Birmingham, *Medical Center*, February 1975, pp. 2–3.

65. A. R. Somers, "Community Health Education: A Challenge to Hospital and Medical Staff," *Journal of the Medical Society of New Jersey*, vol. 70, December 1973, pp. 943-48; A. R. Somers and William Vaun, "What $34,000 Has Done for Long Branch," *Prism*, December 1973, p. 36 ff.

66. P. Cooney, "The New Push in Medicine: Illness Prevention," *Des Moines Sunday Register*, January 12, 1975.

67. American Heart Association, *Cookbook* (New York: David McKay Co., 1973).

68. Chris Imhoff, "DDC—The First 10 Years," *Traffic Safety*, October 1974.

69. E. H. Van Ness, "Address," in *Federal Focus on Health Education: Conference Proceedings*, pp. 9–11.

70. Surgeon General's Scientific Advisory Committee on Television and Social Behavior, *Television and Growing Up: The Impact of Televised Violence* (U.S. Public Health Service, Washington, D.C., 1972), pp. vii, 3-4.

71. Blue Cross Association, "Harris Study Stresses Health Education Need," Chicago, December 29, 1971, p. 16.

72. Lewis and Lewis, "Impact of Television Commercials," pp. 431–35.

73. F. A. Smith, G. Trivax, D. Zuehlke et al., "Health Information during a Week of Television," *New England Journal of Medicine*, March 9, 1972, pp. 516–20.

74. F. J. Ingelfinger, M.D., "Hygeia on the TV Screen," *New England Journal of Medicine*, March 9, 1972, p. 541.

75. C. L. Marshall, M.D., *Toward an Educated Health Consumer: Mass Communication and Quality in Medical Care*, NIH Fogarty International Center, March 1975 (processed), p. 5.

76. Lewis and Lewis, "Impact of Television Commercials," p. 435.

77. B. L. New, M.D., "On the Other Hand," *Medical World News*, March 24, 1975, p. 144.

78. U.S. Congress, Senate, Subcommittee on Communications of the Committee on Commerce, *Hearings on Department of Health, Education, and Welfare's Progress in Developing a Profile on Violence on Television*, 93d Cong., 2d sess., April 1974.

79. *Variety*, January 29, 1975, p. 1.

80. *New York Times*, April 10, 1975.

81. W. H. Kobin, "Encouraging Better Health through Television," *Journal of Medical Education*, February 1975, pp. 143–48.

82. Advertisement for WCVB-TV, *New York Magazine*, November 11, 1974, p. 6.

83. David Victor, "The Role of Television Drama in National Health Education," *Health Education Monographs*, vol. 2, supp. 1, 1974, p. 78.

84. C. L. Marshall, M.D., letter to chairman, April 10, 1975.

85. Earl Ubell, letter to chairman, April 17, 1975.

86. Marshall, *Toward an Educated Health Consumer*, p. 4.

87. H. J. Barnum, Jr., M.D., "Mass Media and Health Communications," *Journal of Medical Education*, January 1975, p. 25.

88. For a useful discussion of the uses and abuses of TV in relation to health education, see God-

frey M. Hochbaum, School of Public Health, University of North Carolina, Chapel Hill, "Motivating People for Better Health," (1974), and President's Committee on Health Education, Task Force on Consumer Health Behavior, Godfrey M. Hochbaum, chairman, *Report*, May 1972 (processed).

89. Surgeon General's Scientific Advisory Committee on Television and Social Behavior, *Television and Growing Up*, p. 210.

90. U.S., Department of Health, Education, and Welfare, National Center for Health Statistics, *Health Resources Statistics*, 1974, p. 139.

91. President's Committee on Health Education, *Report*, p. 27.

92. See Simonds, Appendix F.

93. Donald Campbell, Department of Preventive Medicine, Ohio State University, telephone communication, December 13, 1974.

94. Susan Lee, American Public Health Association, Washington, D.C., telephone communication, December 14, 1974.

95. John Cooper, American Association for the Advancement of Health Education, National Education Association, Washington, D.C., telephone communication, January 2, 1975.

96. Steven Jerritt, American School Health Association, Washington, D.C., telephone communication, December 13, 1974.

97. James W. Dilly, Executive Director, American College Health Association, Evanston, Illinois, telephone communication, January 6, 1975.

98. In 1973 there were 324, 367 active M.D.'s. American Medical Association, *Distribution of Physicians in the U.S., 1973* (Chicago: American Medical Association, 1974), p. 10. In the same year there were 815,000 active registered nurses. *Health Resources Statistics, 1974*, p. 201.

99. *Health Resources Statistics, 1974*, pp. 141–46.

100. *Ibid.*, p. 140.

101. I. S. Shapiro, Ph.D., letter to chairman, April 7, 1975.

102. P. C. Dunn, Ph.D., "An Exploration of the Status and Future Directions of Graduate Programs in Health Education in the U.S.," *Journal of School Education*, vol. 44, November 1974, p. 500.

103. American Medical Association, *Distribution of Physicians in the U.S., 1973*, p. 10.

104. D. M. Blobner, Patient Educator, letter to chairman, February 21, 1975.

105. Richard C. Bates, "Behavioral Medicine Should Be the Next Big Specialty," *Medical Economics*, February 5, 1973.

106. *Health Resources Statistics, 1974*, p. 201. Subtotals are for 1972.

107. H. P. Cleary, D.Sc., telephone communication, April 15, 1975.

108. *Health Resources Statistics, 1974*, p. 245.

109. U.S., Department of Health, Education, and Welfare, Office of the Secretary, Task Force on Prescription Drugs, *Final Report*, Washington, D.C., February 7, 1969.

110. American Pharmaceutical Association, *The Pharmacy as a Health Education Center*, an experimental study conducted by National Analysts, Inc. (Washington, D.C.: American Pharmaceutical Association, 1964).

111. D. A. Knapp, H. H. Wolf, D. E. Knapp, and T. A. Rudy, "The Pharmacist as a Drug Adviser," *Journal of the American Pharmaceutical Association*, NS 9, October 1969, abstracted in Wertheimer and Smith, *Pharmacy Practice*, pp. 373–76.

112. E. E. Madden, Jr., "Evaluation of Outpatient Pharmacy Patient Counseling," *Journal of the American Pharmaceutical Association*, NS 13, 1973, p. 437; J. M. McKenney et al., "The Effect of Clinical Pharmacy Services on Patients with Essential Hypertension," *Circulation*, vol. 48, 1973, p. 1104.

113. See Bass, Appendix H.

114. Imhoff, "DDC—The First 10 Years," p. 35.

115. R. I. Lee, M.D., *A Doctor Speaks His Mind* (1958).

116. Shapiro, letter to chairman.

117. Society of Public Health Educators, "What is a Public Health Educator?" San Francisco, undated.

118. Somers and Vaun, "What $34,000 Has Done for Long Branch," p. 59.

119. *Budget of the United States Government, FY 1975*, p. 119.

120. Kobin, "Encouraging Better Health through Television," p. 144.

121. *Advertising Age*, August 26, 1974; January 6, 1975; November 25, 1974.

122. Alfred McAlister, "Helping People Quit Smoking: Current Progress," in Alan Enelow et al., eds., *Applying Behavioral Science to Cardiovascular Disease* (New York: American Heart Association, 1975).

123. President's Committee on Health Education, *Report*, p. 24.

124. Van Ness, "Address," in *Federal Focus on Health Education: Conference Proceedings*, p. 10.

125. When the health budget of Canada's Department of Health and Welfare is categorized, life style-related expenditures, while still only .1 of 1 percent of the total, rose 278 percent between 1969–70 and 1973–74. By contrast, health care expenditures, which still claim the lion's share, rose only 85 percent. Mark Lalonde, *A New Perspective on the Health of Canadians*, Ministry of National Health and Welfare, Ottawa, 1974, p. 52.

126. J. F. Burnum, M.D., "Outlook for Treating Patients with Self-Destructive Habits," *Annals of Internal Medicine*, vol. 81, September 1974, pp. 387–96.

127. E.g., F. Bass, "A Public Health Approach to Unhealthy Behavior" (Appendix K) *versus* McAlister, "Helping People Quit Smoking."

128. L. W. Green, Dr. P. H., "The Economics of Health Education: Does It Pay?" paper presented to Blue Cross Association Press Seminar, New York City, November 16, 1974 (processed), p. 26.

129. K. Beyers, "Can Health Habits Really Be Changed?" *Prism*, May 1974, p. 13 ff.

130. Stanford University, Institute for Communication Research, *Annual Report 1973–74* (Stanford: Stanford University, 1974), p. 8.

131. J. W. Farquhar, M.D. and P. D. Wood, M.D., cited in "Heart Disease: The Message Gets Across," *Medical World News*, February 10, 1975, p. 8.

132. Marshall, *Toward an Educated Health Consumer*, Summary, p. 5.

133. R. N. Podell, M.D., letter to chairman, March 24, 1975.

134. Kaiser Foundation Medical Care Program, *Preventive Medicine*, Annual Report, 1974 (Oakland, Calif.: Kaiser Foundation, 1974), pp. 19, 21.

135. U.S., Department of Health, Education, and Welfare, Center for Disease Control, National Clearinghouse for Smoking and Health, *Patterns and Prevalence of Teen-Age Cigarette Smoking: 1968–1974*, DHEW Publ. (CDC) 75–8701, Atlanta, July 1974.

136. U.S., Department of Health, Education, and Welfare, National Center for Health Statis-

tics, *Current Estimates from the Health Interview Survey—U.S. 1973*, DHEW Publ. (HRA) 75-1522, Washington, D.C., 1975, p. 6.

137. Peter DelaFlor, New Jersey Cancer Society, telephone communication, January 6, 1975.

138. Don Eddins, Immunization Division, Center for Disease Control, telephone communication, January 6, 1975. Polio immunization among children aged 1 to 4 declined from 73.9 percent in 1965 to 60.4 in 1973.

139. Mrs. Mary Ashley, a member of the Task Force, suggests that financial incentives are essential as "reinforcers" to behavioral change. See Appendix P. For general discussion of motivation in relation to health behavior, see, Hochbaum, "Motivating People for Better Health."

140. Anne R. Sommers, "Consumer Health Education: An Idea Whose Time Has Come?" *Hospital Progress* [Journal of the Catholic Hospital Association], February 1975, p. 10–11.

141. B. A. Rocheleau, *The Technology and Impact of Evaluation in Mental Health Centers in Florida*, University of Florida, Studies in Public Administration no. 33 (Gainesville: University of Florida, 1974), p. 39.

142. President's Committee on Health Education, *Task Force on Consumer Health Behavior*, Hochbaum, chairman, *Report*, p. 67.

143. Blue Cross Association, *A Report on the Health Problems of the Poor* (Chicago: Blue Cross Association, 1968); American Public Health Association, *A Report on the Health Crisis in America* (Washington, D.C.: American Public Health Association, 1970); E. M. Kitigawa and P. M. Hauser, *Differential Mortality in the U.S.* 1973; D. M. Kessner, M.D., *Infant Death: An Analysis by Maternal Risk and Health Care, Contrasts in Health Status*, vol. 1 (Washington, D.C.: National Academy of Sciences—Institute of Medicine, 1973); M. A. Haynes, M.D., "The Gap in Health Status of Black and White Americans," 1973.

144. Editorial, "The Role of Academic Scientists," *Nutrition Action* [Center for Science in the Public Interest], January-February 1975.

145. Earl Ubell, "Health Behavior Change: A Political Model," *Preventive Medicine*, vol. 1, 1972, p. 215.

146. "Report of the Committee for the Assessment of Biometric Aspects of Controlled Trials of Hypoglycemic Agents," *Journal of the American Medical Association*, vol. 231, February 10, 1975. p. 579 ff.

147. "Settling the UGDP Controversy," *Journal of the American Medical Association*, vol. 231, February 10, 1975, pp. 624–25.

148. R. L. Poucher, M.D., AP Story, *Trenton Evening Times*, March 3, 1975.

149. Nearly fifteen years ago, the chairman of this Task Force projected the development of a new type of doctor-patient relationship:

> No single word can adequately describe a complex relationship. Nevertheless, 'educational' may suggest the essence of the newly emerging relationship . . . just as the 'traditionl' relationship is frequently identified as 'authoritarian.' The terms are not mutually exclusive. . . . Yet the differences are fundamental.
>
> Where the authoritarian relationship assumes—and does not discourage—the continued dependence of the patient on the doctor's superior knowledge and wisdom, the educational relationship aims to help the patient understand his illness or problem to assume maximum responsibility for his own recovery, and to overcome his dependence. Where the old relationship was one of unbridgeable inequality, the new is essentially democratic although never quite reaching the point of equality. The doctor remains in full charge of diagnosis and treatment, but makes of his patient an informed, active, par-

ticipant, with full knowledge of the facts and the probable consequences of alternative courses of action. The relationship is basically secular, although it cannot fully dispel the elements of mysticism and faith that overhang the continuing uncertainties and fears surrounding life-and-death situations. H. M. Somers and A. R. Somers, *Doctors, Patients, and Health Insurance* (Washington, D.C.: The Brookings Institution, 1961), pp. 476–77.

150. Podell, letter to chairman, April 15, 1975.

151. L. Breslow, M.D. and C. A. Miller, M.D., *Heal Yourself*, Report of the Citizens Board of Inquiry into Health Services for Americans (Washington, D.C.: American Public Health Association, 1972), pp. 69, 71.

152. An interesting example, from a specialized and very sensitive field, was brought to the attention of the Task Force by Dr. Neil Holtzman, National Academy of Sciences Resident Fellow.

In 1973, the Maryland legislature established an 11 member Commission on Hereditary Disorders of which six members are public representatives. The Commission has the legal responsibility, not only to promulgate rules for the detection and management of hereditary disorders in the state, but also 'to gather and disseminate information to further the public understanding of hereditary disease.' I am privileged to serve on the Commission and believe it is one model for consumer participation and development and oversight of health policy. Letter to chairman, April 9, 1975.

153. Milton Terris, M.D., "Breaking the Barriers to Prevention: Legislative Approaches," *Bulletin of the New York Academy of Medicine*, vol. 51, no. 1, January 1975, pp. 242–57.

154. A. M. Schmidt, M.D., "The Role of Regulation in Educating the Public about Health," *Journal of Medical Education*, vol. 50, February 1975, pp. 124-29.

155. Fred Bass, M.D., letter to chairman, April 22, 1975.

156. E.g., A. R. Somers, *Health Care in Transition: Directions for the Future* (Chicago: Hospital Research and Educational Trust, 1971), p. 85; President's Committee on Health Education, Task Force on Consumer Health Behavior, Hochbaum, chairman; *Report*, President's Committee on Health Education, *Report*.

157. National Health Council, "Preliminary Report on the Development of a Plan to Establish a National Center for Health Education," New York City, March 1, 1975 (processed).

Part III
Summary and Recommendations

MAJOR FINDINGS

Consumer health education (CHE) in the United States today is, like so many other institutions in this rapidly changing society, at a crossroads, philosophically and programmatically. The dogmas of the relatively quiet past are clearly no longer adequate to the turbulent present and the uncharted future. No one is entirely sure of the correct road to the future. But, again to paraphrase President Lincoln, if we would know whither we are tending, we must know whence we came and how we got here.

Throughout Part II we have tried to summarize the major recent developments in health education and related fields and to identify the principal issues and problems, not in order to belittle the past but to help lay the foundation for a new and reinvigorated future. These issues and problems, as we have noted from the beginning, are both internal and external. The following are among our major findings and conclusions:

1. A New Definition of Consumer Health Education

The following definition was unanimously adopted by the Task Force: The term "consumer health education" subsumes a set of six activities that—

1. inform people about health, illness, disability, and ways in which they can improve and protect their own health, including more efficient use of the delivery system;

2. motivate people to want to change to more healthful practices;

3. help them to learn the necessary skills to adopt and maintain healthful practices and life styles;

4. foster teaching and communications skills in all those engaged in educating consumers about health;

5. advocate changes in the environment that will facilitate healthful conditions and healthful behavior; and

6. add to knowledge through research and evaluation concerning the most effective ways of achieving these objectives.

Obviously, not every CHE program has to take on all six functions. But any organization or institution, that aspires to leadership in the field must be committed to the full range. In particular, we rejected as "health education" any program that is limited to dissemination of information and does not involve efforts at behavior change where needed. Great stress was also placed, at the present stage of development, on the incorporation of research and evaluation in all major programs.

2. Consumer Responsibility

There is increasing evidence of a significant, positive relation between the following: an informed responsible consumer attitude toward preventive care and health maintenance, responsible patient adherence to prescribed regimens, and a responsible sense of participation in health care policy decisions affecting both individual and community health.

To emphasize the importance of the consumer's own role, we deliberately chose the term "consumer health education" for the name of the Task Force and the title of our report, although in the interest of brevity, we continue to use the older term "health education" interchangeably.

3. Major Categories

Six major types or categories of health education program were identified: patient education, school health education, occupational, community, national, and media programs. While there is obvious overlap between some of these categories, there is also a general distinction in terms of target audience, sponsorship, institutional setting, professional input, methodology, and financing. For analytical purposes it was convenient to think in terms of these major subdivisions. Federal funding programs should probably recognize some, but not all, of these distinctions.

4. Consumer Health Education as a "Field of Interest"

Health education programs are being carried on today not only by specialists in health education but by physicians, nurses, dentists, media specialists, and members of a broad range of additional professions and occupations identified with the fields of health, education, communications, and the new "consumerism." Health education is not a single discipline but a "field of interest," drawing on knowledge from the biomedical, biostatistical, and behavioral sciences as well as on various administrative, planning, and research skills.

Numerous disciplines and would-be disciplines are involved. It is not now possible to say which will emerge as dominant a decade hence. All should be encouraged, but all should be continuously and critically evaluated. None should be taken for granted.

5. A Field in Transition

The best word to describe the philosophy and practice of health education today is "transitional." On the positive side, there is one very important factor: the tremendous vitality associated with the field. This vitality is reflected in the exciting variety of programs, in the multiplicity of professions and occupations now involved in one way or another and reflected, for example, in the membership of this Task Force, in the gradual rise in available funds, and in the growing amount of serious research and evaluation. These achievements, in the face of overwhelming obstacles, are to be warmly applauded.

But there are also many shortcomings, and, if CHE is to achieve its potential, they must be recognized and corrected. Among these are imprecision and/or lack of agreement as to goals, definitions, and methodologies; the vast array of fragmented, uncoordinated, and often duplicating programs in some communities alongside the almost total absence of programs in others; the inadequate number of trained full-time educators; the marginal commitment of most of the other professions and occupations; the inadequacy of training even for most of the full-time people; the lack of sufficient understanding of individual motivation in the health field and consequently of how to help people adopt more healthful behavior; and numerous difficulties with respect to research and evaluation.

6. Inadequacy of Current Funding

Current funding levels are grossly inadequate by every measure applied: comparison with total U.S. health care expenditures, the federal health budget, individual hospital budgets, the cost of individual programs, and—most dramatically—by comparison with the advertising budgets of over-the-counter drugs. For example, the manufacturer of a single product, Alka-Seltzer, spent in 1975 about seven times as much to promote its use as the entire budget of the federal Bureau of Health Education. CHE expenditures, as a percentage of national health expenditures or individual hospital budgets, are in the order of ¼ to ½ of one percent.

7. Effectiveness

While the effectiveness of CHE as a whole is widely debated, there is now evidence from a number of studies that well-designed programs, incorporating the various elements of CHE included in our definition, can be effective in producing desired behavior change if accompanied by national policies and mass communications programs designed to reinforce, rather than undermine, the educational goals.

8. Interrelationship of Health Education and Health Promotion

CHE cannot succeed in an environment where national health policy and the allocation of national health resources are keyed almost exclusively to health care (the diagnosis and treatment of illness and disability) and where major policies in related areas such as agricultural subsidies, food assistance, product advertising, housing, and law enforcement, that impact directly on the health of the people, are frequently in direct conflict with recognized health goals.

At the same time, even a favorable external environment is unlikely to result in significant progress in CHE unless the field itself is greatly strengthened. Hence the two major interrelated thrusts of this report: health promotion and consumer health education.

Consumer health education is not synonymous with health promotion. It is only one of several strategies by which a general policy of health promotion is carried out. In keeping with the charge to Task Force IV, however, it is the area to which we devoted primary attention.

RECOMMENDATIONS

The recommendations that follow are presented in very general terms. No effort has been made to achieve detailed specificity. Our aim is to achieve as broad a consensus as possible on the general goals. Once this has been achieved, the additional work needed to translate general goals into specific legislative proposals or other instruments of implementation should not be too difficult.

The recommendations are presented in three parts. Recommendations 1 and 2 are concerned with overall policy. Without agreement on these basic matters, it is impossible to develop meaningful implementation strategies. Such agreement is essential to provide a consistent basis for federal and state legislation, manpower development, financing, evaluation, and many other purposes.

Recommendations 3–11 are concerned with implementation of an effective national strategy of consumer health education. They are designed to strengthen the field by a broad program of public and private support for the various categories of CHE, aimed at the development of recognized and stable disciplines that could be expected to carry out a strengthened mandate.

Recommendations 12–13 deal with the external obstacles. They attempt to establish a framework for implementation of a meaningful national commitment to health promotion, a general policy umbrella under which the field of consumer health education and the various disciplines operating therein may be expected to develop their maximum potential.

Since Task Force II on Environmental Health is addressing itself to the general problem of occupational health, our Task Force is making no recommendations in this area. This should not be construed as indicating lack of interest or concern. On the contrary, we believe that the workplace constitutes an important educational site for instruction about nonoccupational as well as occupational health problems. The employment relationship also frequently provides a valuable incentive to positive behavior change.

Recommendation 1 — Health Promotion

The nation's basic health policy, recognized by both public and private sectors, should be health promotion, involving, in balanced proportion, all the means or strategies subsumed under the definition of promotion: research, education for the health professions, public health, environmental protection, occupational health, consumer health education, health care (diagnosis and treatment of illness and disability), and health economics (organization and financing). The official statement of mission, organization, and functions of the Assistant Secretary of Health should be restated to include specific responsibility for all aspects of health promotion as here defined.

Despite the impressive advances in medical science and medical technology during the past half century, despite the rapid rise in the proportion of national resources being devoted to health care in the United States, and despite the estimated $118.5 billion we are spending on health care in FY 1975, our health indices remain unsatisfactory. In some respects, such as death rates for young and younger middle-aged men, these indices actually worsened during the sixties. The major causative factors relate far more to the environment and to individual behavior and life style than to health care as such.

It now appears that therapeutic medicine, important as it is, has reached a point of diminishing returns. Clearly the time has come for a basic rethinking of national health priorities. The time has come to transfer some meaningful proportion of national health resources to strategies other than health care, the most expensive of all the strategies and the one that has been allowed to monopolize resources during the past few decades.

The intent is not therapeutic nihilism. The intent is a better balance, more closely related to actual individual and national health needs.

A number—perhaps most—of the essential components of an effective health promotion capability are already present in the health side of the Department of Health, Education, and Welfare, especially the Center for Disease Control, the Food and Drug Administration, and the Office of Drug Abuse Prevention. Many of the activities carried on in the three other major operating bureaus—Health Resources Administration, Health Services Administration, and the National Institutes of Health—are concerned with health promotion in one form or another. Consumer health education is the most important single omission, which we propose to correct through creation of a new Office of Consumer Health Education (Recommendation 10).

Even with the addition of this new office, however, we still feel that the whole would be less than the sum of the parts. There is still need for more explicit emphasis on promotion, prevention, and consumer education to guide the Assistant Secretary for Health in determining priorities and in allocating resources and as a symbol of reorientation of national priorities away from the now uncontrollable costs of health care to the more cost-effective preventive programs.

Recommendation 2 — Consumer Health Education

Consumer health education, as defined in this report, requires major new emphasis throughout the public and private sectors. The federal government has a special responsibility, related to both economic and health factors, to provide the essential leadership, including the channeling of adequate national resources into CHE research and programs.

To be fully effective, the various health promotion strategies must be interrelated. For example, it is now clear that even the most advanced and sophisticated health care system is ultimately dependent for effectiveness on informed and motivated patients and other consumers. At the same time, it is clear that no consumer health education strategy can succeed without the active cooperation and support of physicians, nurses, and other health care professionals actually involved in patient care.

In view of the overriding importance of individual behavior and life style as major factors in the nation's unsatisfactory health status and ever-rising health care bill, CHE, with its emphasis on education and motivation of the individual and better individual use of the delivery system, must now be recognized as a top priority in the national commitment to health promotion.

Health education of the total population should be initiated in early childhood, when basic patterns of life style and health-related behavior are being established. It should also be continued throughout life, changing with the changing needs of the individual and keeping pace with new health information and practices. As a long-term goal for allocation of resources to health education, the Task Force adopted a target figure of 6 percent of national health expenditures.

Effective implementation of this policy will call for multiple initiatives on the part of all concerned—including the health professions, schools of health professions, hospitals and other health facilities, the school systems, organized labor and industry, other consumer groups, all the mass media, the drug and appliance industries, and state and local governments. However, the federal government, with its Constitutional commitment to the national health, its unparalleled resources and potential for leadership, and its ever-growing health care bill, must be prepared to assume the leadership in developing this new priority.

Recommendation 3 — Provider Requirements

Require, as a condition of federal, state, and local funding, that all hospitals, HMOs, neighborhood health centers, and other community health facilities—both public and private—provide consumer health education, as defined in this report and in regulations to be promulgated by the Secretary of Health, Education, and Welfare, as an integral part of their service responsibilities to their individual users and to their service constituencies.

The need for a specific locus of responsibility for both patient and community health education is clear. So is the intimate relationship between patient education and patient care. While other institutions, e.g., state and local health departments, medical schools, and university extension services are, in some areas, operating useful programs, the Task Force felt that, for the nation as a whole, hospitals and other health care institutions provide the most practical and nearly universal site for fixing responsibility.

In thousands of communities throughout the country, the hospital or other care institution is the only place where the patient or community health educator can find a reliable base of operations and the necessary backup resources.

Moreover, although many hospitals still construe their role primarily as "the doctor's workshop" rather than a "community health center," the leadership of the hospital industry and the more progressive institutions are moving in the latter direction—a move that the Task Force felt should be encouraged. Hospitals now engaged in both patient and community education report a sometimes unbroken continuum between activities designed for the inpatient, the outpatient, and asymptomatic health care consumer living in their service areas. The challenge, we felt, was to persuade the hospital industry as a whole to assume responsibility for such a continuum.

To assure quality, some form of professional and/or agency quality review should be required, although at first the standards should be few and basic only, to avoid the kind of difficulties now faced by many HMOs as a result of too rigorous federal standard setting.

Further, in the case of nonpatient or community programs, special steps should be taken to assure that the program is actually addressing community needs and to avoid unnecessary duplication. To this end, each facility should submit a community health education plan for review by the local and/or regional health planning body (Recommendation 7) or its delegate agency.

Federal requirement of a specified amount of health education, for example as a condition of participation in Medicare, would help greatly to raise the status of CHE within the institutional hierarchy and resource-allocating mechanism. Such a requirement could be met either through special organized programs, or through the activities of individual members of the professional staffs, or, ideally, by a combination of both.

One method would be to express the requirement as a percentage of the institutional budget, varying by type of institution. For a hospital, for example, the first year requirement might be only .5 of 1 percent, rising to 1 percent in the second year, 1.5 percent in the third, and gradually moving up to 5 or 6 percent. For a neighborhood center or other primary care institution the proportion would be much higher.

Recommendation 4—Third-Party Reimbursement

Require or encourage all third-party payers—public and private—to reimburse providers for the net costs of patient education.

Third-party reimbursement is both an essential and practical means of stimulating institutional commitments to patient education. Without some such regular and reliable source of funding, it is difficult to see how patient education can ever achieve the quality and status essential to effective performance.

Fortunately, a number of the major private health insurance carriers and plans, including the Blue Cross Association and the Health Insurance Association of America, are committed to the concept of patient education and third-party reimbursement therefor. HMOs are required to provide health education programs as a condition of federal planning and development grants. It is difficult, however, in view of the necessity for competitive pricing for plans or carriers, to implement such a commitment on an individual basis. The general lack of adequate coverage for ambulatory care is also a major obstacle to routine reimbursement.

All carriers and plans should now be encouraged, through federal and/or state policy, to include patient education for both inpatients and outpatients as a covered benefit.

In particular, the federal government should take the lead by amending the Medicare and Medicaid laws to include health education programs, as defined by the Secretary of Health, Education, and Welfare, as reimbursable items and by stipulating specific coverage in any national health insurance legislation or other major extensions of existing financing programs.

Recommendation 5—School Health Education

Encourage coordinated, comprehensive school health education programs through federal research and development funds and grants-in-aid to states.

Federal funding is needed in three areas: developing and evaluating school health education curricula, training teachers in health education, and encouraging state education agencies to take a more active role in promoting school health education.

Many school systems interested in implementing comprehensive school health education programs are inhibited by the lack of acceptable, coordinated curricula and the high costs of developing their own. Federal research and development funds should be made available to state and local educational agencies for the development and testing of appropriate curricula, with particular attention to the special needs of the poor and members of minority groups, taking into account the frequent needs of these groups to adapt to a culture and a language foreign to their own.

There is also a serious shortage of adequately trained school health educators. Federal funds should be used to evaluate and upgrade training programs, to train larger numbers of educators, and to encourage the inclusion of health education in the training and continuing education of general classroom teachers.

State education departments are the primary overseers of public school districts. Except in a few states, they have neglected health education. Federal grants-in-aid should be used to encourage more active consideration and participation. In particular, they should be resource centers for school health education activities throughout their states.

Finally, the Task Force deplores the traditional barriers that exist between our education and health "systems." There is a pressing need for stronger and more effective linkages between the two.

We welcome introduction of the Meeds-Clark bill (H.R. 2599 and S. 544) into the 94th Congress, as addressing several of these major concerns.

Recommendation 6—Research And Development

Provide federal support for research and development in consumer health education techniques, methodologies, and programs, and their evaluation.

Despite the considerable number of significant CHE programs scattered across the country and the efforts of thousands of dedicated professionals, the general "state-of-the-art" is in need of much greater precision and development. The program of public and private support recommended in this report must be accompanied by intensive efforts directed to improvement of health education definitions, principles, techniques, and methodologies and to the formulation of more precise criteria and protocols for both implementation and evaluation, including criteria for patient education by individual diagnosis.

In brief, the entire field requires greater discipline. This effort should include a rigorous assessment of the state of the art and delineation of areas of strength and weakness in knowledge, looking toward development of a national statement of priorities and realistic goals.

Much of the support, as well as initiative, for these efforts should come from the private sector. But there is a special need for federal leadership. Federal support, with special emphasis on evaluation, should be made available to qualifying institutions, organizations, and agencies in all six categories of CHE—patient education, school health education, occupational, community, national, and media programs.

We note the existence of a number of community "laboratory" populations for the study of problems in health and/or education. Such communities should be encouraged to participate in the development and evaluation of health education methodologies. We also endorse the development of large-scale programs, such as the Stanford Heart Disease Prevention Program, specifically designed to test health education hypotheses.

Closely related is the need for expansion of the present valuable surveys and studies of the National Center for Health Statistics to include more information on consumer health status, health behavior, and related data useful not only in planning, but also in evaluation of, health education programs and techniques. Relevant resources of the Center for Disease Control should also be fully explored and utilized.

Recommendation 7—Systems, Networks, And Centers

Provide federal support for the development of regional and state systems or networks of consumer health education programs as well as one or more national "centers" in the private sector.

Even with the severely limited funds and personnel now available for CHE, there is considerable duplication and waste. Still more important, most American communities lack access to any comprehensive consumer health education.

To avoid these inefficiencies, to promote optimum utilization of both money and manpower, and to help develop a stable infrastructure for community and other programs, it is highly desirable to develop local, regional, and/or state networks. This can be accomplished through the coalescence of existing programs, new regional and statewide initiatives under the leadership of a state health department, a university extension system, a state hospital or professional association, a medical school, regional medical program, or other organization with the concern and resources to play the coordinator role, or through a combination of various approaches. Consideration should also be given to combining CHE and continuing professional education in a single state or regional network.

The National Health Planning and Resource Development Act of 1974 (P.L. 93–641) provides a potential mechanism for promoting such networks. We have already proposed, in Recommendation 3, that each hospital or other facility, reimbursed for its health education programs through federal financing, be required to submit a community health education plan for review by the appropriate local and/or regional planning body. Under the new law, such plans could be coordinated through the Health Systems Agencies (HSAs) and the State Health Planning and Development Agencies and special funds could be made available to the states for development of the proposed networks. Insofar as possible, resources of the Center for Disease Control should also be utilized for this purpose.

We commend the National Health Council for leadership in attempting to develop a "National Center for Health Education" in the private sector. While we do not believe that any one organization has yet demonstrated its capacity to speak for all the varied interests and groups that are currently or potentially active in CHE, it is logical that the National Health Council, building on the historic interest of its member organizations, should play a responsible leadership role. This should not preclude the establishment of additional national or regional "centers" as other groups emerge with demonstrated capabilities.

Recommendation 8—Media Programs

Call on the leadership of the television and advertising industries and appropriate representatives of the public to help television achieve its full potential as a major national resource for consumer health education through two separate but related approaches: (a) the two industries should establish a Council on TV and Consumer Health Education to assume leadership in developing a long-range industry-wide plan for health education programming and funding; and (b) the federal government, through the appropriate responsible agencies—DHEW, the Federal Communications Commission, and the Federal Trade Commission—and the television and advertising industries, especially the proposed industry council, should intensify their efforts to find voluntary solutions to the complex issues of health-related product advertising and the currently unacceptable levels of violence in programs directed primarily to children and general family viewing. The three agencies should report to the Senate and House Subcommittees on Communications before July 1, 1976. If, by that time, no substantial progress has been achieved in the opinion of the chairmen of those subcommittees, we request Congress to consider establishment of some permanent review mechanism for children's and family TV, consisting of appropriate public, professional, and industry leaders. No additional regulatory authority is requested.

The impact of television as an informational and motivational force in contemporary U.S. society, especially in relation to children and individuals with less-than-average schooling, can hardly be exaggerated. With respect to health-related behavior, it is difficult to say, today, whether the net impact has been positive or negative.

The positive can be documented by a growing list of first-rate health documentaries, public service "spots," and even some of the theatrical programs presented by the Public Broadcasting System and the three commercial networks. The negative has been convincingly documented by a number of carefully designed professional studies including two prestigious national commissions looking into the relationship between televised violence and individual behavior.

Despite this Jekyl and Hyde record, the Task Force believes that, with more consistent and accountable attention from the leadership of the industry, with more high-level assistance from representatives of the public and the health and education professions, and with identification of adequate sources of financing for constructive programs, the postive potential can be greatly enhanced and the negative minimized.

Our emphasis on TV is by no means intended to belittle the influence of the press, radio, and other media that have also produced some excellent material and whose continuing participation should be enlisted in the national effort to improve consumer health education. Since TV's capacity for both positive and negative impact is so crucial, however, we think the primary effort, at the present time, should be aimed in this direction.

The purpose of part "a" of Recommendation 8 is to mobilize the resources of television and advertising in the development of a long-range, multiaudience, multiformat series of programs, utilizing documentaries, theatrical programs, cartoon and news programs, public service spots, and all other appropriate formats, aimed at helping the American people increase their understanding of, and ability to cope with, health and health-related problems. Both commercial and public TV should be involved. Assistance in funding through public and private sources should be explored. The existence of such a formally designated industry council would also provide a body to which the public and the health and education professions could relate.

The Task Force is aware that the National Advertising Council shares many of our concerns, and we hope it will play an important role in relation to the proposed new council. The Advertising Council, however, is not designed to carry out the kind of concentrated systematic health education program we are calling for. Nor is it adequately representative of the television industry.

The purpose of part "b" of Recommendation 8 is to encourage the television and advertising industries, the DHEW, including the Food and Drug

Administration, the FCC, and the FTC to intensify their efforts—through voluntary advertising codes, "family viewing hours," and other means—at effective self-regulation. The "review mechanism," if established, should not be given powers of censorship. However, the committee would be expected to make use of fact-finding publicity, nongovernmental sanction, and all the moral and political force it could command to secure elimination of material deemed, by objective professional opinion, to be injurious to the nation's health.

Recommendation 9—Health Education Manpower

Request the Secretary of Health, Education, and Welfare to arrange for the conduct of a study or studies of consumer health education manpower to determine current and future needs for all categories and levels of personnel and to recommend appropriate education and credentialling policies.

Both quantitative and qualitative improvements in CHE manpower are essential if the national efforts recommended in this report are to be effectively implemented. As a first step, we recommend a high-level Departmental review of personnel in all the extensive varieties noted in this report. Such a review would apply not only to health education specialists but to all the health and related professions currently involved in some aspect of health education and should address itself to the numbers and types needed, their preparation, accreditation, distribution, and continuing education.

Special attention should be given to the introduction and development of health education concepts and methodologies into basic education for the various health professions, including medicine, dentistry, nursing, pharmacy, and public health. The time is ripe for such a new initiative. Witness the special attention paid to health education at the 1974 annual meeting of the Association of American Medical Colleges and the fact that most state nursing practice acts now specifically mandate patient education as a routine aspect of nursing care. Explorations, looking to increased health education content, are now in order with the AAMC, the American Medical Association, the Coordinating Council on Medical Education, the National Board of Medical Examiners, the American Dental Association, the American Pharmaceutical Association, the American Nurses Association, National League for Nursing, the Association of Schools of Allied Health Professions, the National Commission for Accrediting, and other professional organizations.

For health education specialists, studies are needed in cooperation with the Society of Public Health Educators (SOPHE), the American Public Health Association, American School Health Association, American College Health Association, and related groups. For these professions, special efforts are needed to determine the numbers of students required at entry levels, bachelor's, master's, and doctor's levels, as well as the types of educators needed in the schools, health care institutions, industrial settings, community agencies, national health agencies, and the media, and the need for special research personnel and future teachers.

Finally, we urge that the new task force give special attention to the definition and development of a new occupational category of indigenous community health education aides, advocates, or facilitators to act as a bridge between the community, especially in low-income areas, and health providers, including health educators. The success of programs utilizing such individuals, under various names, has been demonstrated in a number of locations, but the concept needs more precise definition, more standardized training, and some form of academic certification. The possibility of utilizing funds available under temporary public service employment programs emphasizes the need for immediate attention to this area. However, the need is by no means confined to periods or areas of high unemployment, and the program should be seen as a permanent aspect of a comprehensive community health system.

Whatever format the study assumes, it should be given high visibility and provide adequate opportunity for general public input.

Recommendation 10—DHEW Office of Consumer Health Education

Establish a high-level Office of Consumer Health Education in the Department of Health, Education, and Welfare with adequate status, authority, and other resources to carry out the various federal responsibilities and duties recommended in this report.

Among these responsibilities are the following:

A. formulation of national goals, strategies, and priorities for consumer health education and general responsibility for their implementation;

B. oversight of the requirement that all hospitals and other federally funded health care institutions provide a specified amount of CHE and that federal funding, planning, and quality assurance programs be made compatible with this requirement (Recommendations 3, 4, and 7);

C. oversight of the national CHE research, development, and evaluation program, including related activities of the Center for Disease Control and the National Center for Health Statistics (Recommendation 6);

D. financial and technical support to states and other public and private agencies and organizations in the establishment of state, regional, and/or national networks and centers and continuing exchange of information and cooperation with such programs (Recommendation 7);

E. liaison with the communications media (Recommendation 8);

F. cooperation with the study of long-range financing proposed in Recommendation 11 and oversight of the disbursement of revenues raised in accordance with Congressional action following such study;

G. help in establishing and staffing the Task Force on Health Education Manpower (Recommendation 9) and in implementation of its recommendations.

In addition, the Office of Consumer Health Education should be the focus of staff responsibility and work with the Secretary and Assistant Secretary in the monitoring of federal programs and policies with significant impact on individual health status (Recommendation 12) and for advocacy of the health education point of view vis-a-vis competing interests.

Among the major resources available to the proposed office would be a high-level Consumer Health Education Advisory Council, representative both of professionals and consumers knowledgeable in the various areas of consumer health education.

The optimum location for an Office of CHE is debatable. The most obvious place is in the Office of the Assistant Secretary for Health, but most important is that the new office be positioned wherever it can be assured of maximum financial and political support.

Establishment of the proposed new office under the Assistant Secretary implies no criticism of the Center for Disease Control (CDC). There are many areas related to the operational aspects of CHE where CDC's technical and programmatic assistance and its impressive network of regional and state experts in disease prevention and control could be very useful. The new office and the state networks, proposed in Recommendation 7, should be specifically instructed to work with CDC in this respect. Special funds for this purpose are suggested in Recommendation 11.

Recommendation 11—Financing

Request the Congress to (a) authorize two-year funding in the order of $100 million to carry out the programs and functions proposed in this report; and (b) commission a study of long-term CHE financing by The Brookings Institution or some equally competent research organization.

How much would it cost to carry out the recommendations proposed in this report? It is impossible to say with precision. Four—1, 2, 4, and 13—are simply statements of policy and carry no special price tag. Any additional cost involved in the implementation of Recommendation 4—third-party payments for patient education—would be met through those institutions, it is hoped, in part through economies on patient care. The proposal for school health education research and development—Recommendation 5—we assume would be met through separate legislation, such as the Meeds-Clark bill.

We have set a tentative figure of $40 million (first year) and $60 million (second year) for the cost of the remaining recommendations—those that involve the new Office of Consumer Health Education (OCHE) and its numerous functions, including those taken over from the old Bureau of Health Education (BHE); financial support for various new research and development projects; promotion of CHE networks, centers, and media programs; regulatory and review functions; the special Task Force on Health Education Manpower; and additional functions requested of the National Center for Health Statistics and the Center for Disease Control.

In arriving at these figures we have tried to reconcile the competing claims of a noninflationary federal budget and the necessity of providing at least enough financial support to give the new program a chance of succeeding. Major elements of the projected $40 million first year might include:

	(in millions)
DHEW-OCHE start-up and basic operating costs, including assimilation of present functions of BHE	$5.0
Additional regulatory and review functions	2.0
Task Force on Health Education Manpower	.5
Additional funds for National Center for Health Statistics	3.0
Additional funds for Center for Disease Control	1.5
Extramural grants and contracts	
5 large scale basic research programs @ $1 million each	5.0
8 academic centers @ $250,000 each	2.0
20 state networks @ $500,000 each	10.0
National Center (National Health Council)	1.0
4 experimental TV series @ $2 million each	8.0
Other R and D projects	1.0
Miscellaneous	1.0
	$40.0

The estimated cost of the basic research programs is related to the cost of the successful Stanford Heart Disease Prevention Program—over $750,000 for first year (1970) and $4 million for five years. The cost of the state networks is derived in part from the experience of the College of Medicine and Dentistry of New Jersey.

The media projection is far less than the cost of the PBS's "Feeling Good," $7 million. The National Center figure is that requested by the National Health Council under pending Congressional proposals.

The principal factor in the $20 million increase projected for the second year would be the addition of thirty more state networks—$15 million.

With respect to the long-term costs, including those that would be met through third-party payments, school budgets, voluntary agencies, and so forth, the Task Force has set a tentative goal of 6 percent of total national health care expenditures. Obviously, we need a much more precise figure as well as a timetable for moving from the present ¼-½ of 1 percent toward 6 percent and a study of alternative methods of financing. For example: Should the financing of CHE be closely related to that of national health insurance? How much reliance on social security taxes, on general revenues? Should there be special taxes on cigarettes, alcohol, and other health-threatening products? Should there be special taxes on certain nonprescription drugs where overuse or other abuse is common?

Because of its recognized competence in both fiscal policy and health economics, we suggest The Brookings Institution conduct such a study. We would hope that the study could be completed within a year.

Recommendation 12—Health Impact Reviews

Request the Secretary of HEW and the Assistant Secretary for Health to undertake immediate and continuing review of major federal policies and programs impinging on individual, community, and national health and, wherever determinations are made that the impact is harmful, to recommend corrective action to the President, other Departmental heads, and/or Congress, as appropriate.

Areas that should come under such continuous monitoring include agricultural supports for harmful products, such as tobacco, or those potentially harmful if used to excess, such as beef with high fat content; school lunch and food assistance programs; food and drug advertising; speed limits; and other energy conservation measures. The conflicts or apparent conflicts between a number of existing programs in these areas and the goals of health promotion have been increasingly publicized in recent years.

The monitoring should extend not only to areas where harmful or allegedly harmful policies now exist but to those currently marked by the general absence of essential health promotion policies, including low-income housing, the control of violence, and public service employment. The anomaly of spending billions of federal dollars to patch up the victims of big city violence, squalor, and frequently intolerable living conditions while refusing to face up to the root causes cannot be indefinitely sustained as general economic conditions deteriorate, budgetary constraints increase, and various safety valves disappear.

Individual Task Force members have prepared or introduced proposals or statements dealing with several of these issues including the prevention of atherosclerotic heart disease, hypertension, better nutrition education for school children and other especially vulnerable groups, approaches to the control of violence, and financial incentives as a reinforcer for health education (Appendices G, M, N, O, and P). Some aspects of these statements have been dealt with in earlier recommendations; some go beyond the charge to our Task Force. However, we commend all five to the attention of the National Conference on Preventive Medicine, the Congress, the Administration, the health professions and all concerned with the health of the American people. These issues should be high on the priority list to be reviewed by the Secretary of HEW and his staff.

We are aware that policy development in all these areas cuts across Departmental lines and that DHEW can do little or nothing alone. We feel strongly, however, that the Department should be continuously engaged in monitoring such policies, in advising the President, the Congress, and the American people with respect to such policies, and in representing the health point of view in intradepartmental decision making. Primary responsibility for staff work should be lodged in the proposed Office of Consumer Health Education.

The importance of DHEW involvement in broad policy issues, beyond the usual definition of health and medical care, was emphasized both by the Surgeon General's Committee on Smoking and Health and the subsequent Committee on Television and Social Behavior. Some would have preferred to see strong recommendations included in their reports. But, even without recommendations, the carefully documented findings emerging from such a prestigious source have been useful.

In initiating such a large new undertaking, an essential first step would be establishment of a list of long-term goals and short-term priorities and some mechanism for subsequent alteration in the lists. Criteria, both immediate and long run, should include the firmness of the presumptive causal relationship between the policy—or nonpolicy—in question and national health status, the financial cost to the nation of failure to take corrective action where needed, and the reasonable possibility of corrective action.

For example, in the case of tobacco, the causal relationship between cigarette smoking and health has been professionally and offically determined; the health care costs resulting from cigarette smoking are known to be enormous—currently estimated by the National Center for Health Statistics at $11.5 billion a year; and some corrective action, while difficult, has not proved insuperable, at least with respect to one form of advertising. The Surgeon General acted reasonably a decade ago in allotting top priority to this area. It is now high time to follow up by addressing the problem of public subsidies to tobacco growers and higher taxes on cigarette consumption.

A second example might be gun control. Homicide and suicide are now among the leading causes of death in the United States. Within the 15–24 age group, they are the second and third leading causes, exceeded only by accidents. Approximately two-thirds of all murder victims are killed with guns, and this proportion increased steadily throughout the sixties. The number of handguns in the United States today is reported to be 40 million, rising by 2.5 million each year.

The cost of health care for the victims of shootings plus the cost of law enforcement to protect against more shootings, is obviously very high. Corrective action has thus far proved extremely difficult. To our knowledge, however, no effort has been made to enlist the support of the health professions in pressing for new policies in this area. Under leadership of the Secretary of HEW, this support could make the difference.

In determining priorities for health policy review, the Secretary should be prepared to exercise great flexibility. In the highly volatile U.S. socioeconomic climate, new dangers and new opportunities present themselves almost daily. It would be futile to try to alter priorities with each such change in the environment. But it would be equally foolish to ignore major new developments.

For example, the current extensive unemployment not only presents new difficulties for health maintenance and health care financing but also presents new opportunities for public service employment. A massive public service effort, especially in the hard-pressed construction industry, could well be directed to a major war on urban and rural slums and squalor. The enlistment of unemployed youths in such a war could produce four positive results: more and better housing for low-income families at lower cost, skills for the unskilled, reduced crime, and improved health status.

While some may claim that Recommendation 12 goes beyond the province of the National Conference on Preventive Medicine as well as Task Force IV, the majority feel that the time has long passed when the health care field—one of the largest employers in the nation, one of the major consumers of national resources, and a major source of national inflation—can continue to maintain an aloof posture on such issues. Responsible preventive action requires that we take a stand and lend our support, at all levels of policy formulation, to their correction.

Recommendation 13—Public-Consumer Participation

Urge the Secretary of HEW and Congress to take immediate steps to develop more, and more effective, public-consumer participation in the development and oversight of health promotion policies at all levels of policy making, from the Office of the President to local hospital and PSRO boards.

Provider domination of the current U.S. health care delivery system is obvious, understandable, and—perhaps to some extent—inevitable. The results have not been entirely negative. Dedicated physicians, scientists, dentists, nurses, pharmacists, hospital administrators, and other professionals have helped to raise the standards of U.S. health care and to extend the accessibility of care to most of the population. But the negative results are now becoming clearer, not only in such egregious faults as have been revealed in some segments of the nursing home industry but, more fundamentally, in the apparently uncontrollable inflation and the increasing disparity between resource allocation and the nation's major health problems.

Domination by consumers, most of whom lack knowledge of the technical aspects of health promotion, would probably be equally unproductive. A balance of provider and consumer interests is needed. By definition, the Congress and the Secretary of HEW are expected to represent the public interest. Even with the best intentions, however, they are unable to monitor effectively all the manifold health programs. Effective consumer input is needed at all levels to assure meaningful public accountability.

We realize that the mere presence of a substantial number of consumers, however defined, on a policy-making body will not automatically assure such accountability. Recent experience has revealed a number of problems with consumer participation. For example, statutory requirements for majority consumer representation on federally funded planning bodies have not produced any dramatic changes in the behavior of such bodies.

The reasons, however, remain to be identified; we believe, first, that many are correctable. Second, we are not advocating rigid or arbitrary quotas that, if carried to extremes, could obviously render a decision-making body inoperable. Third, we believe that input from consumers is needed not only to assure them a voice in health resource decisions, but—equally important—to help develop a sense of responsibility with respect to the use and abuse of health resources and maintenance of their own health.

Concepts of consumer participation vary from a single ombudsman or patient representative employed by a hospital, to majority representation on decision-making boards. The purposes, methods, and values obviously vary widely. For our purposes—development of the broadest possible base of well-informed, motivated, and responsible health care citizenship—we recommend, in addition to the Advisory Council to the proposed Office of Consumer Health Education (Recommendation 10):

A. establishment of a National Advisory Committee on Health to report directly to the President, with equal representation of providers and consumers, both to be chosen for knowledge of the industry;

B. requirement, as a condition of federal funding, of significant proportions of knowledgeable consumers on all state, regional, and local health institutions and agencies, including hospital, nursing home, and PSRO boards, HMOs, planning agencies, etc.

C. requirement, as a condition of participation in federal programs, of significant proportions of knowledgeable consumers on the boards of all health insurance carriers or intermediaries participating in Medicare, Medicaid, and other federal funding programs, including national health insurance, if and when enacted.

Appendix A
Witnesses and Guests—Task Force Meetings

WITNESSES: CHICAGO, NOVEMBER 13–14, 1975

Stanley S. Bergen, Jr., M.D.
President
College of Medicine and Dentistry
  of New Jersey

Joseph A. Bryk, Ph.D.
Senior Research Associate
National Safety Council

Donald Campbell, Ph.D.
Department of Preventive Medicine
Ohio State University

Congressman William S. Cohen
2nd District, Maine
(Represented by Cynthia Hilton,
  Legislative Assistant)

Gerald J. Driessen, Ph.D.
Research Coordinator
National Safety Council

Joy G. Dryfoos
Director of Planning
The Alan Guttmacher Institute
Planned Parenthood Federation of America

Donnell Etzwiler, M.D.
Director
Diabetic Education Center
Minneapolis, Minnesota

John Farquhar, M.D.
Department of Medicine
Stanford University School of Medicine

Herbert K. Gatzke
Director
Bureau of Manpower Education
American Hospital Association

Rosalind Hawley
President
Core Communications in Health, Inc.
New York, New York

Donald J. Merwin
Director
National Center for Health Education Project
National Health Council

Philip Morgan
Program Director
Training and Community Programs
Office of Consumer Health Education
College of Medicine and Dentistry of
    New Jersey

Horace Ogden
Director
Bureau of Health Education
Center for Disease Control
Department of Health, Education, and Welfare

Lewis C. Robbins
Executive Secretary
Health Hazard Appraisal
Methodist Hospital of Indiana

Leonard Rubin, M.D.
Coordinator of Education
Kaisar Permanente Medical Group

James Schoenberger, M.D.
Chairman, Department of Preventive Medicine
Rush Presbyterian Hospital—St. Luke's
   Medical Center
President, Chicago Heart Association

Keith Sehnert, M.D.
Department of Community Medicine
   and International Health
Georgetown University School of Medicine

Lloyd A. Shewchuk, Ph.D.
American Health Foundation
New York, New York

William Vaun, M.D.
Director of Medical Education
Monmouth Medical Center

Sidney Wolfe, M.D.
Director
Health Research Group

OTHER GUESTS: TASK FORCE MEETINGS

Dr. Emile Bendit
Alcohol, Drug Abuse, and Mental
   Health Administration
DHEW
Parklawn Building
Rockville, Maryland 20852

Mr. Donald Carmody
Director
Division of Health Protection

Office of Policy Development & Planning
OASH-DHEW
Parklawn Building
Rockville, Maryland 20852

Mr. Edward Friedlander
Special Assistant
Office of the Commissioner
Food and Drug Administration
DHEW
Parklawn Building
Rockville, Maryland 20852

Mr. J. Larry Fry
Acting Deputy Minister of Health
Department of National Health and Welfare
Brooke Claxton Building
Ottawa, Canada

Ms. Cynthia Hilton
Legislative Assistant to Congressman
    William S. Cohen
Longworth Building, Room 1223
Washington, D.C. 20515

Dr. Neil Holtzman
Institute of Medicine
National Academy of Science
2101 Constitution Avenue, N.W.
Washington, D.C. 20418

Mr. Terrance Keenan
Vice-President for Grants Management
Robert Wood Johnson Foundation
The Forrestal Center
Princeton, New Jersey 08540

Ms. Nancy LeaMond
Division of Health Protection
Office of Policy Development & Planning
OASH—DHEW
Parklawn Building
Rockville, Maryland 20852

Ms. Mona Mitnick
Office of the Assistant Secretary for
  Planning and Evaluation
DHEW—North Building
Washington, D.C. 20201

Douglas Niblett, M.D.
Director General
Community Health Service
Department of National Health and
  Welfare
Brooke Claxton Building
Ottawa, Canada

Dr. Harrison Owen
National Heart and Lung Institute
National Institutes of Health
Building 31, Room 5A10B
Bethesda, Maryland 20014

Dr. Kent Peterson
The Association of University
  Programs in Hospital Administration
1 Dupont Circle
Washington, D.C. 20007

Ms. Dorothy Rice
Social Security Administration
Office of Research and Statistics
1875 Connecticut Avenue, N.W.
Washington, D.C. 20009

Ms. Elsa Schneider
Office of Education
Division of Drug Education
DHEW — FOB 2043
Washington, D.C. 20201

Dr. Arthur Viseltear
Subcommittee on Health
Dirksen Senate Office Building, Room 4220
Washington, D.C. 20510

Appendix B
Federal Health Budget—FY 1975

HEALTH
(In millions of dollars)

Program or agency	Outlays			Recommended budget authority for 1975[1]
	1973 actual	1974 estimate	1975 estimate	
Development of health resources:				
Supporting biomedical research..........................	1,639	2,035	2,188	1,964
Training health manpower...	712	693	776	428
Proposed legislation..........	.....	5	20	20
Constructing health facilities.............................	188	264	216	.....
Improving the organization and delivery of health services......................	244	349	184	128
Proposed legislation..............	.....	.....	40	75
Subtotal, development of health resources........	2,784	3,345	3,424	2,615
Financing or providing medical services:				
Financing medical services:[2]				
Medicare (trust funds).....	9,479	12,180	14,191	16,714
Medicaid...........................	4,600	5,827	6,563	6,592
Proposed legislation......	.....	.....	-55	-55
Other financing....................	849	1,057	1,264	1,218
Providing medical services...	345	430	430	413
Proposed legislation......	.....	.....	42	42
Health insurance for Federal employees.............................	17	-12	-23	.....
Subtotal, financing or providing medical services........................	15,290	19,482	22,412	24,925
Prevention and control of health problems:				
Preventing and controlling diseases..............................	203	239	213	244
Consumer safety....................	143	206	237	243
Subtotal, prevention and control of health problems........................	346	445	450	487
Deductions for offsetting receipts:[3]				
Proprietary receipts from the public......................	-4	-4	-5	-5
Total.............................	18,417	23,268	26,282	28,022

[1] Compares with budget authority for 1973 and 1974, as follows: 1973, $22.226 million; 1974, $26,153 million.

[2] Entries net of offsetting receipts.

[3] Excludes offsetting receipts which have been deducted by subfunction above: 1973, $1,860 million; 1974, $2,507 million; 1975, $2,846 million.

Source: U.S., Office of Management and Budget, *The Budget of the United States Government, Fiscal Year 1975*, p. 119.

Appendix C
Health Education in The Mid–70's— State of the Art

by
Scott K. Simonds, Dr. P.H.*

INTRODUCTION: PHILOSOPHY AND SCOPE

The ultimate goal of health education is the improvement of the nation's health and the reduction of preventable illness, disability, and death.[1]

Human behavior is recognized as being a direct cause of or at least a significant contributor to both health and illness, as well as being a critical factor in the control and treatment of disease. Health education is that dimension of health care which is concerned with influencing behavioral factors and is therefore complementary to those components of health care that are concerned more with the organic factors of health and disease. As such, health education is a vital and indispensable component of health care delivery in which virtually all health professions must be involved.

The purpose of health education is to bring about behavioral changes in individuals, groups, and the larger populations from behaviors that are presumed to be detrimental to behaviors that are presumed to be conducive to present and future health.

In this, health education activities may address themselves to specific behaviors such as nutrition, immunization, family planning, prenatal care, or compliance with medical regimens. But in the long run, health education of the public aims at more general, basic, and lasting changes in people's life style and daily living practices by endowing children and adults with a sense of value of health and a sense of responsibility for their own health, as well as with the will and capacity to discharge this responsibility persistently and conscientiously within the limits of their ability.

In order to achieve its purpose, the tasks of health education are not only to inform people about health and disease and ways in which they can protect and improve their health, and to motivate people to want to change to

*Director of Health Education Programs, University of Michigan School of Public Health Ann Arbor, Michigan; Member of Task Force on Consumer Health Education.

more healthful practices, but also to enable them to adopt and maintain healthful practices.

The goal of knowledgeable and motivated consumers of health services has been pursued generally through processes and means of communication and education in the traditional sense. However, even in the presence of requisite health knowledge and motivation, the adoption of healthful practices is often inhibited or rendered impossible by social, economic, situational, and other conditions in people's living environments. It is recognized that appropriate changes in such environmental conditions may produce changes in people's health behavior that even the most effective educational efforts alone are unable to bring about. Health education in its broader context, aimed as it is at actual behavioral change, addresses itself purposefully to these conditions as well as to the more traditional and narrower targets of improving people's health knowledge, attitudes, and motivation. Thus health education encompasses activities carried out with, through, and by those agencies and organizations which play key roles in the country's economic, political, health, and other social systems as well as through many professional disciplines.

FROM EARLY DEVELOPMENTS TO CURRENT PRACTICE

The roots of health education have been traced to the early Greek period, but as an emerging profession, health education is generally considered to have begun in the United States in 1919 when the term was first used at a conference of the Child Health Association or in 1921 when the first graduate fellowship was awarded for study in health education.

The art and science of health education have been fairly consistent with and parallel to the state of the knowledge on which it was based at any one point in time. Early practice, while based on philosophy, theory, research, and practice in education, journalism, group work, and community organization, gradually incorporated developing knowledge from the social sciences, particularly field theory, and from studies of communications. The advances in the social sciences since the late 1950s have had a profound effect on health education and are considered to be the scientific foundations of current practice. As theory has developed in the social sciences, health education benefited in terms of redefinition of the conceptual stance. Centers for advanced study in health education all place great emphasis on the social sciences, with particular concern for applications from psychology, social psychology, sociology, anthropology, and political science and their relation to health behavior, behavior change, and organizational change.

Emerging from such centers is an increasingly socioecological view of behaviors of individuals, groups, and communities which are seen as resulting from the interaction of multiple forces. Because health behaviors result from complex interacting forces and are rarely the result of one force per se, health education concerns itself with planned change and broad social interventions as well as direct methods with individuals, families, and groups.

The simplistic model of change that suggests that behavior is modified by merely providing information has long since given way to a systems view that suggests that change may occur as the result of knowledge growth, but that attitude and behavior changes may not automatically follow, and, in fact, the order may be reversed. A host of studies based on the knowledge-attitudes-practice (so-called KAP studies) have not proven to be very useful in the design of planned change, and much research is needed to understand how and under what conditions and with what populations planned communication may induce behavior change.

EMERGING DIRECTIONS

Health education has emerged in the mid-1970s as one part of more comprehensive interventions and approaches to social change.[2] It is increasingly recognized that there must be far more change in the environment to support health behavior and far more social and environmental reinforcement for changes encouraged. The frequency with which individuals are found to have adequate knowledge but do not take appropriate actions suggests that problems in health education are related more to linkages between knowledge and action than to knowledge per se. A belief model that incorporates cognitive elements which are linked to motivations to act has promise of providing additional support for communication approaches to behavior change. In addition, however, increasing concern is found for social support systems and social networks as linkages and reinforcers for the individual, and as channels of communication to special populations. Although research in group work and community organization has slowed in recent years, there remains great support for findings from earlier research and from the current philosophy of consumer activism and for individuals being increasingly involved in making decisions that affect their lives. Indeed, the whole notion of the activated consumer and the activated patient suggests that a key focus of health education is the enhancement of skills to enable individuals to take matters into their own hands increasingly—to shape their own destinies, and to shape their environments to meet their needs. This further suggests that more attention must be given to changing the health system to meet the needs of individuals, rather than limiting the use education as a way of "adapting" individuals to the system, which so frequently occurs, and for increasing attention to health education "outreach" programs.

These emerging trends in consumerism and increasing rejection of "person blame" psychologies indicate that health education during the mid-1970s will be concerned with such themes as health education as social policy, health education as related to social and organizational change, and comprehensive approaches to the field of health education itself.

NOTES

1. Discussion in this section is derived from National Health Council, preliminary draft, "Materials for Summary of Proceedings," Conference on Functions of the National Center for Health Education, Chicago, December 4–5, 1974; and President's Committee on Health Education, Task Force on Motivation, Godfrey Hochbaum, chairman, *Report on Motivational Behavior*, Washington, D.C., May 1972 (processed).

2. Discussion is this section is derived from Marshall Becker, ed., "Personal Health Behavior and Health Belief Model," *Health Education Monographs*, vol. 11, no. 4, 1974; Snehendu Kar, "Communication Research in Family Planning: An Analytical Framework," paper prepared for UNESCO, March 1974; Scott K. Simonds, "Health Education As Social Policy," *Health Education Monographs*, vol. 2, supp. 1, 1974, pp. 1–10; and Scott K. Simonds, "Considerations for the Design of a Comprehensive Health Education Delivery System," in *Papers on Theoretical Issues in Health Education*, Dorothy Nyswander International Symposium, Berkeley, California, September 1974, pp. 173–183.

Appendix D
St. Francis Medical Center
Trenton, New Jersey
Consumer Health Education

| | Year Ending December 1974 | | | | | |
Patient Programs	Hrs. per course	No. of times repeated	Total Hrs.	No. of Participants	No. of Instructors	Teaching Format*
1. Mothers Classes	1½	116	174	940	1	D
2. Prenatal Classes (Cln.)	1	52	52	252	1	D
3. Expectant Parents	6	3	18	170	4	D-F (Tour, Film)
4. Diabetes Classes (Cln.)	1	84	84	85	2	A, C, D
5. Cardiac Patient Educ.	- -	92	- -	92	- -	A, D, F (Film)
6. Heart Club	2+	13	26	18	2+	A, D (Group)
Community Programs						
1. Employee Health Semrs.	1	34	34	508	1	D, F (Film)
2. Smoke-No-More Program	16+	1	16+	40	6	D, F (Film)
3. "Diabetes & You"—Sr. Cit.	2	2	4	91	1	D, F (Film)
4. "Hypertension & You"—Sr. Cit.	1	1	1	110	1	D
5. Diab. Youth On Tar. (DYOT)	2½	16	24+	30	4	D (Group)
6. Parents of Diab. Teens	3	1	3	10	2	D
7. Alcoholism Series	1	2	2	203	2	D, F (Film)
Inservice Programs						
1. Learning & Teach. Prin.	8	1	8	32	4	D
2. Diabetes in Older Pat.	1½	4	6	38	1	D, F (Film)
3. Cardiac Instruc. Orient.	2	8	16	123	3	A, D
4. Diabetes Instruc. Orient.	1	7	7	90	1	D, F (Film)
5. Diabetes Seminar	½	1	½	20	1	D
Conferences						
1. Learn & Teach. Prin. (RMS)	8	1	8	35	3	D
2. Cardiac PT. Ed. (Ht. Assn.)	3	1	3	33	1	D
3. St. Francis School of Nursing	2	2	4	70	1	D, F (Slides)

2787 Subtotal

Health Screening & Education					
1. Hypertension	(May)	2	5	10	216
2. Pap Smear	(June)	5	1	5	325
3. Glaucoma	(Sept.)	2	1	2	150
4. Health Carnival	(Oct.)	7	1	7	1655 (3000+)
5. Diabetes	(Nov.)	4	1	4	385
6. Hypertension—Sr. Cit.	(Dec.)	2½	1	2½	86

2817+ Subtotal

5604 Grand Total

*A. Individual instruction
B. Closed circuit TV program
C. Lecture with simulation (e.g., skill practice)
D. Lecture with discussion
E. Self-instruction
F. Other

Appendix E
Health Education in the Primary Care Setting

by
T. Franklin Williams, M.D.*

In my view, every primary health care setting—health maintenance organizations, group practices, individual practices through some referral arrangement—should be expected to provide for their clients or patients systematic educational programs, first, of a general health maintenance and preventive nature, and second, disease-specific education for anyone with an identified chronic illness or propensity to such an illness.

Furthermore, persons enrolled for or receiving their primary care in any setting should be expected to participate in such educational activities. Audit review should include evaluation of their participation as well as evaluation of the educational programs offered. Reports of such audits should be presented, first of all to the individual patient and secondly to the governing or advisory body concerned with the primary health care system in which the patient is enrolled, which in most and perhaps all instances will include representatives of the consumers enrolled.

This point of view in effect carries the "contract" approach a step further: the health provider agrees to provide systematic patient education and the patient agrees to do his part in this educational process. This might best be written into the contract signed by the patient when he signs up with a given primary care program or insurance arrangement.

Such educational services themselves may often best be provided through some common efforts serving a number of primary care settings, depending upon the size and diversity of such settings. A large prepaid group practice might provide its own program in all respects. Smaller groups or partnerships and individual practitioners might need to be able to refer their patients to patient education services or centers developed in hospitals or other settings to provide these specific services.

*Professor of Medicine, University of Rochester School of Medicine and Dentistry; Medical Director, Monroe Community Hospital, Rochester, New York. This appendix is an excerpt from a letter to the chairman, March 18, 1975.

111

I have just (March 17, 1975) visited an excellent example of such a hospital-based patient education center for ambulatory diabetic patients at the Women's College Hospital in Toronto, a combined effort of that hospital plus Mount Sinai and Toronto General Hospitals to provide such a service for patients referred by practitioners throughout the Toronto area, financed by the provincial government. Dr. George Steiner of the University of Toronto and Mrs. Elizabeth Laugharne are best informed about that program.

The Board of the American Diabetes Association has endorsed the position I have described above for diabetes patient education; its Committee on Diabetes Education Centers and Systems of which I am now chairman has the responsibility to develop proposed standards for such patient education services, which it is hoped would be accepted as qualifying such services for reimbursement for costs in both public and private health insurance systems.

Appendix F
Health Education Manpower

by
Scott K. Simonds, Dr. P.H.*

Although health education and professionally trained health educators have been a part of community health services since 1922, there is no single source of valid data on health education manpower. The report of the President's Committee on Health Education cited that there were "25,000 professional health educators—persons with degrees (bachelor's to doctoral) in either school or community health education,"[1] when, in truth, there is not a valid statistical basis for the figure.

A review of the literature shows that published health education manpower research has been undertaken primarily by Rosemary M. Kent in a longitudinal study to determine annual numbers of students, graduates, and active workers in public health education since 1944.[2] Elena M. Sliepcevich has documented the institutions offering programs of specialization in health education at the undergraduate and graduate levels and in schools of public health.[3] The American Public Health Association has made available data on numbers of graduates of programs in public health education in schools of public health accredited by APHA and has provided other relevant data arising from committee reports, usually unpublished. Other existing data appear to be estimates of personnel employed in health education work as determined and reported by professional organizations including the Society for Public Health Education, American School Health Association, and the American Alliance for Health, Physician Education, and Recreation. Other published sources of incidental or relative information have come from divisions of the U.S. Public Health Service, doctoral disserations, and testimony before the President's Committee on Health Education.

Since no single source of data is available, the problem of evaluating, reconciling, and using accurately the potentially conflicting statistics becomes great.

*Director of Health Education Programs, University of Michigan School of Public Health; Ann Arbor, Michigan; Member of Task Force on Consumer Health Education.

CURRENT SUPPLY AND LOSSES

Kent has estimated the current supply of personnel, trained in schools of public health or other APHA accredited programs in community health education at the master's level and beyond and who are employed in public health education work as something under 1,100.[4] Attrition, for whatever reason, is accounted for in this estimate. Another estimate is 2,000 to 3,000, a figure cited as being provided by the Society for Public Health Education.[5] This latter estimate probably takes into account personnel trained in health education at the master's level or beyond from schools of public health or APHA accredited programs, as well as other institutions.

An Ad Hoc Task Force on Professional Health Manpower for Community Health Programs, convened in 1973, projects the current supply of professional employed public health educators at 2,000.[6] The Task Force based its projection on the estimate of 1800 health educators having graduated from accredited master's-level programs up to 1970.[7]

Estimates on currently available personnel trained at the bachelor's level or beyond with a major specialization in health education in a setting other than a school of public health are virtually nonexistent. Most persons trained in such programs enter school health education work. An estimate of the number of school health educators employed in 1971 was 20,000,[8] but the statistic is not documented and likely includes persons employed in school health education who have not been prepared in that field. The American Alliance for Health, Physical Education, and Recreation has reported approximately 4,000 members as citing school health education as their primary field,[9] out of a total organizational membership of around 30,000.

The American School Health Association reported 8,000 members who were school health educators in 1971,[10] but similarly this group also includes personnel trained in nursing and other disciplines.

The figure of 25,000 professional trained health educators cited earlier is a "guestimate" at best, and is based on organizational memberships perhaps more than anything else.

In all likelihood, a better estimate of the total number of individuals prepared in health education at the baccalaureate, master's, or doctoral levels and working actively in the field of either public health education or school health education would be no more than 12,500 and those prepared on community or public health education would accont for no more than 2,000 of this total. In any case, it is clear that a more definitive study of health education manpower is needed than has been done.

PROJECTED REQUIREMENTS

The earliest projections for health education manpower were made in 1945 in the Haven Emerson Report[11] in which one health educator (presumably MPH or MSPH trained) was recommended for each 50,000 population in local health department units. The criteria for the projection were related to the service setting and some sort of "service load" among nurses, sanitarians, and other professional personnel in the unit. If that criteria were applied today, there should be approximately 4,320 health educators in local health departments. The number currently so employed is unknown, but generally believed to be no more than one-quarter of these projected requirements.

Additional estimates have been made more recently ranging from recommendations of one health educator per 9,000 to one per 25,000, although again there is a lack of a clear rationale for these ratios. The Division of Manpower Intelligence, Department of Health, Education, and Welfare, has estimated a need for 4,000 professionally trained health educators by 1980 beyond those 2,000 estimated to be presently employed.[12]

The manpower projection of a total of 6,000 public health educators required by 1980 was likely made in the absence of knowledge about major developments in the health sector which will make further demands on professional prepared manpower, such as the following:

● the movement in hospitals (7,000 member hospitals of the American Hospital Association) toward increased programming efforts in personal and community health education;

● initiation of reimbursement procedures so that health care facilities can be reimbursed for patient education services by third-party payers;

● inclusion of health education within the legislation for health maintenance organizations;

● inclusion of health education as a basic function of regional health systems;

● potential inclusion of health education within national health insurance legislation.

It is likely, therefore that the figure of 6,000 is an underestimate.

Although no adequate assessment of existing vacancies exists for health education manpower, it is evident from a recent study of job offerings in *Journal of the American Public Health Association* that health educators at the MPH/MSPH level are among the most frequently sought-after professionals.[13]

A forthcoming publication on health education manpower,[14] indicates that serious gaps exist in present knowledge about health education manpower and that new studies must be undertaken. The need to look at health education tasks performed by other disciplines and increasing use of health education manpower trained at baccalaureate levels for first-level positions are but two of the major developments in the field itself affecting total requirements. New groups of educators within the health care systems, such as diabetes educators, indicate that the health and patient education function is spreading rapidly in the health care system. New kinds of health education manpower are being considered for positions in hospitals and other health care facilities.

NOTES

1. President's Committee on Health Education, *Report*, Department of Health, Education, and Welfare, 1973, p. 18.

2. Rosemary M. Kent, "Public Health Educators: Manpower Today and the Changing Scene," *Journal of the American Public Health Association*, vol. 59, no. 6, 1969, pp. 1003–42.

3. "Institutions Offering Programs of Specialization in Health Education," Elena M. Sliepcevich, director, *School Health Education Study*, Washington, D.C., January 1970.

4. Rosemary M. Kent, "Professional Public Health Education National Manpower," testimony before President's Committee on Health Education, Atlanta, January 27, 1972.

5. U.S., Department of Health, Education, and Welfare, National Center for Health Statistics, *Health Resources Statistics, 1972–73*, p. 159.

6. Ad Hoc Task Force on Professional Manpower for Community Health Programs, Thomas L. Hall, coordinator, *Professional Health Manpower for Community Health Programs*, Department of Health Administration, School of Public Health, University of North Carolina, Chapel Hill, 1973, p. 52.

7. Ibid.

8. *Health Resources Statistics, 1972–73*, P. 159.

9. Ibid.

10. Ibid.

11. Haven Emerson, *Local Health Units for the Nation* (The Commonwealth Fund, 1945).

12. U.S., Department of Health, Education, and Welfare, Public Health Service, National Institutes of Health, Bureau of Health Manpower Education, Division of Manpower Intelligence, *Provisional Estimates*, Washington, D.C., 1972, p., 73.

13. Ad Hoc Task Force on Professional Manpower for Community Health Programs, Hall, coordinator, *Professional Health Manpower for Community Health Programs*, p. 121.

14. Scott K. Simonds, Robert Bowman, and Deanna Mechensky, "New Directions for Health Education Manpower Studies" (forthcoming).

Appendix G
Violence and the Health of American Youth

by
Philippa Chapman*

In 1973, 17,800 young Americans ages 15 to 24 died in motor vehicle accidents;[1] 4,162 were murdered;[2] and 4,098 committed suicide.[3] The three main causes of death for young Americans in this age group are all violent.

Death is the most measurable effect of violence, yet for every youth killed in a car accident, hundreds are injured, maimed, or incapacitated. Similarly, for every murder victim, scores are victims of aggravated assault and rape. For a significant proportion of American youth, violence is a major health problem; for an alarming number it is a matter of survival. The causes and prevention of violence must be considered in any analysis of means to improve the health of the nation's youth.

As growing affluence has made automobiles and motorcycles more accessible, the young have increasingly been both victims and agents of traffic accidents. Motor vehicle accidents in 1973 accounted for 46.2 deaths per 100,000 population, a 16 percent rise from 1963.[4] In 1973, persons under 25 constituted 21.7 percent of the nation's drivers but caused 36.3 percent of the nation's fatal accidents and 39.4 percent of all accidents.[5] Seven hundred thousand persons under 25 were injured in motor vehicle accidents in 1973.[6] The rise in popularity of motorcycles among young people has added to youthful fatalities; motorcycles produce four times as many fatalities per vehicle mile as do other vehicles.[7] The number of automobile injuries could be decreased considerably by the enforcement of auto safety features and the 55 miles-an-hour speed limit, which, since its implementation, has already lowered the death toll where it has been enforced.[8]

When one bears in mind that numerous auto deaths, listed as accidental, are considered by many experts to be suicides, the already significant problem of youthful suicides becomes even more serious. In 1973, the suicide rate for those 15 to 24 was 10.6 persons per 100,000 population. The rate has more than doubled between 1950 and 1973.[9] In Los Angeles County, where

*Research Assistant

117

careful suicide statistics have been kept, the youthful suicide rate has more than doubled in the last ten years.[10] In 1972, for all ages combined, the sex difference in suicide rates was larger than the race difference. White males are two and one-half times as likely to commit suicide as white females; black males are almost five times as likely to commit suicide as black females.[11]

VIOLENT CRIME

Not only is there an alarming increase in the number of young people who inflict violence on themselves, but there is also a dramatic increase in the number who inflict violence on others. Violent crime, particularly in the city, is concentrated especially among youth. Rates of arrest for urban homicide are much higher for the 18 to 28 age group than for any other. Moreover, it is in these age groups that the largest increases have occurred. There was also a dramatic 300 percent rise in assaults between 1958 and 1967 for those in the 10 to 14 age group.[12]

There is evidence of a substantial rise in youthful murders of strangers and of interracial victims.[13] In 1973, 6,616 people 15 to 29 were murdered,[14] indicating that the victims generally have the same youthful characteristics as the offenders. In the cities, victimization rates are generally highest for young males, poor persons, and blacks.[15]

The problem continues to accelerate. Between 1960 and 1973, there was a 160 percent increase in the number of violent crimes per 100,000 population;[16] an 86 percent rise in the number of murders.[17] By 1973, there were 9.3 murders per 100,000.

The death rate from homicide is characteristically highest for those 25 to 29. The age group born in 1953–57, the last years of the high postwar birth rate, will be in the 25–29 age bracket in 1982. Therefore, it must be feared that, unless the upward trend in homicide is reversed, the homicide death rate will continue to rise at least until that time.[18] The increase is such that it has been estimated that 2 percent of all babies born in the larger American cities will probably be murdered eventually, and the actual figure might reach as high as 5 percent.[19] This is the average risk; it varies according to race and sex. For example, in 1972 for all ages combined, mortality from homicide among nonwhite males was ten times greater than among white males, while the rate among nonwhite females was six times the rate among white females.[20]

The lack of legislation requiring gun control has meant that there were, in 1968, an estimated 90 million guns in circulation,[21] weapons which not only make possible many accidental shootings but have been increasingly used in violent crime. The number of aggravated assaults and armed robberies increased from 15 percent in 1967 to 21 percent in 1972. Similarly, an increasing number of murder victims are killed by guns; in 1964 the proportion was 55 percent; in 1972 it was 65.6 percent.[22]

If any immediate reduction in violent crime is to be achieved, the control of arms and ammunition must be a high priority at all levels of administration in this country.[23] Although this is obviously a political issue involving special interests, gun control legislation could have a marked effect in reducing homicide. A recent analysis of the efficacy of state and municiple controls on handguns concluded that many lives would be saved if all states increased their level of control to that of New Jersey.[24]

The greatest increase in homicide has been at ages 1–4.[25] This increase indicates the more accurate recording of deaths from child abuse as a result of greater awareness of the problem—the "battered-child syndrome."[26] However, systematic information on physical abuse of children continues to be scarce; the nature and full scope of the phenomenon are uncertain.[27] One upper estimate concluded that, nationwide, 50,000 children could be expected to die annually and 300,000 to be permanently injured through maltreatment.[28] The physical abuse of children results in serious, often irreversible, damage to their physical well-being and emotional development. These abused children may, in turn, be more prone to abuse their children and commit violent behavior.[29] David G. Gil suggests,

> To the extent that American society may succeed in reducing the amount of violence and abuse which it inflicts collectively on children in the course of their socialization, it may reduce the amount of violence in interpersonal and intergroup relations among adults in this country, and perhaps even in international relations on a global scale.[30]

Conversely, violence in the international arena may lead to an acceptance of violence as a method of solving personal problems. The prolonged involvement of the United States in the Vietnam War is considered by some to have brutalized many Americans.

> The experience of war over a long period devalues human life and habituates people to killing . . . . When violence is legally sanctioned for a cause in which people see no moral purpose, this is an obvious stimulus to violence for what they may maniacally consider moral purposes of their own.[31]

TV AND VIOLENCE

Yet the Vietnam War was obviously only one of the many influences in recent American life that can help to explain the pervasiveness of violent behavior in youth. Both the National Commission on the Causes and Prevention of Violence (1969) and the Surgeon General's Advisory Committee on Television and Social Behavior (1972) analyzed the possibility that the prevalence of violence on television leads to violent behavior in youth.

The commission did not conclude that television was a principal cause of violent behavior in society. It saw violence on television as only one factor, but an important, contributing one.

> We believe it is reasonable to conclude that a constant diet of violent behavior on television has an adverse effect on human character and attitudes. Violence on television encourages violent forms of behavior, and fosters moral and social values about violence in daily life which are unacceptable in a civilized society. . . . It is a matter for grave concern that at a time when the values and the influence of traditional institutions such as family, church, and school are in question, television is emphasizing violent, anti-social styles of life.[32]

Among the commission's recommendations was one to the TV networks to reduce the amount of violence on their programming and to conduct their own research.

> It is time for them to stop asserting "not proved" to charges of adverse effects from pervasive violence in television programming when they should instead be accepting the burden of proof that such programs are not harmful to the public interest.[33]

The commission also recommended that parents take responsibility for supervising their children's viewing.

The Surgeon General's Scientific Advisory Committee on Television and Social Behavior was initiated at the request of Senator John O. Pastore, Chairman of the Senate Subcommittee on Communications, who was concerned about TV violence and its possible social consequences. Although the committee was composed of "recognized experts in the behavioral sciences and mental health disciplines," the television industry was permitted to, and did, exercise a veto over several proposed members.[34] The Secretary of HEW also determined that the committee would confine itself to "scientific findings" and make no policy recommendations.

Research for the two-year study was carried out under supervision of the National Institute of Mental Health through independent projects subject to the usual NIH review procedures. Clinical experiment focused on the effects of TV violence on child behavior, while surveys inquired into the violence viewing of young people and their tendencies toward aggressive behavior.

The carefully, almost tortuously, worded summary reflects the divergent interests involved in the study:

> There is a convergence of the fairly substantial experimental evidence for *short-run* causation of aggression among some children by viewing violence on the screen and the much less certain evidence from field studies that extensive violence viewing precedes some *long-run* manifestations of aggressive behavior. This convergence of evidence constitutes some preliminary indication of a causal relationship, but a good deal of research remains to be done before one can have confidence in these conclusions.[35]

These conclusions aroused considerable dispute, almost immediately, as some committee members felt the summary underemphasized the dangers revealed in the scientific studies.[36] The committee itself urged the serious student to examine the five volumes of background reports and papers published concurrently with the final report.[37]

Senator Pastore has since held two sets of hearings to clarify and publicize the report and to find out what progress the networks have made toward reducing the violence in their programming.[38] The first hearing was held in March 1972.[39] As a result, the committee recommended that the Department of Health, Education, and Welfare and the Federal Communications Commission jointly develop a method of measurement of TV violence.

In opening the second hearing in April 1974, Senator Pastore stated that the Surgeon General's committee had unanimously concluded, "The causal relationship between televised violence and anti-social behavior is sufficient to warrant appropriate and immediate remedial action."[40] The prestigious five member Science Research Committee set up by HEW and FCC to conduct a feasibility study of a violence profile has as yet made no formal report.[41]

The impetus has now shifted to the FCC. Chairman Wiley has met with the network presidents, who also testified at the hearings, to remind them that they were expected to make some progress in this area. With the networks' cooperation, the concept of a "family viewing hour" was developed.[42] The networks have agreed to this self-regulation. NBC stated its policy as follows:

> Violence will be shown only to the extent appropriate to the legitimate development of theme, plot, or characterization. It should

not be shown in a context which favours it as a desirable method of solving human problems, for its own sake, for shock effect, or to excess.[43]

The National Association of Broadcasters Television Code has now been amended to include the concept of a "family viewing hour."[44]

The impact of television and the media in general remains controversial.[45] There is as yet no clear evidence of cause and effect, but there are very few who now claim that there is no relationship between televised violence and actual violent behavior.[46]

UNDERLYING SOCIOECONOMIC CAUSES

Society has changed with unprecedented speed since World War II. Cohesiveness and stability in the local community have declined as has the extent to which parents are able to provide children with a standard of morality coinciding with the mores of the larger society. This is particularly true in urban areas.

For many young people, their peer group rather than the family, school, or church, has come to dictate their behavior. Demographically, the "youth cohort" is also a larger proportion of the population, so that, even apart from the erosion of traditional authority, the "baby boom" youth are supervised by fewer older adults than in previous generations. Many young people are unable to communicate with their families and feel isolated and unloved. For those unable to participate in society because of unemployment or lack of skills, the propensity for violence is greatly increased.

> To be a young, poor male; to be undereducated and without means of escape from an oppressive urban environment; to want what the society claims is available (but mostly to others); to see around oneself illegitimate and often violent methods being used to achieve material gain; and to observe others using these means with impunity—all this is to be burdened with an enormous set of influences that pull many toward crime and delinquency. To be also a Negro, Puerto Rican, or Mexican-American and subject to discrimination and segregation adds considerably to the pull of these criminogenic forces.[47]

We have little precise knowledge of the social, economic, and psychological variables associated with many of the youthful accidents and violent deaths; therefore they are difficult to prevent. We do know, however, that violent crime is overwhelmingly an urban phenomenon. The twenty-six cities with 500,000 or more residents and containing about 17 percent of our total population contribute about 45 percent of the total reported violent crime.[48]

The causal relation between crime and urban life is tied in with other social and health problems. Crime rates are highest in the poorest areas of the city, areas characterized by physical deterioration, declining population, high density, economic insecurity, unemployment,[49] poor housing, family disintegration, transiency, conflicting social norms, and an absence of constructive positive agencies.

Physical decay, coupled with poverty and family disintegration, seems to infect people with a tendency toward violent antisocial outlets for their deep-seated difficulties. All too often, the "other outlets" are narcotics or alcohol. The rising number of teenage alcoholics is another aspect of the drug problem that has serious consequences for health and is a cause of many, if not most, teenage automobile accidents. The heroin epidemic that broke out in 1963 and 1964 reached its peak in 1969 or 1970 seems to be related to the violent behavior of youth, particularly violent assaults by youth, although the data do not permit the conclusion that the increased use of heroin led, in and of itself, to a comparable increase in crime.[50] Drug overdoses may also account for some of the increase in the suicide rate.

CONCLUSION

If there is no one cause for the epidemic of violent behavior among young Americans, there is certainly no simple solution. Violence is widely acknowledged to be a serious problem, but there are also widely divergent approaches to policy in this area.

Some claim that American youth has lost its sense of responsibility, that it has been spoiled by affluence, and what it needs is stricter discipline in homes, schools, and church, stricter penalties for those committing violent crimes (to be enforced by a more powerful police force), and the return of the death penalty for those committing homicide. Others say that violence is learned and for youth it is a sign of frustration and rejection; therefore the epidemic is not going to be stopped by punitive measures. Since society is responsible for creating the conditions that lead to violent crime, these conditions must be modified if youthful violence is to be abated.

The propensity for self-destructive behavior in increasing proportions is often seen as a sympton of alienation in American youth. The feeling of youthful alienation is perhaps one of the most insoluble problems in this society, and this might remain the underlying malaise unless the priorities of the country change significantly. At least a partial solution would be provided by reforming the education system and encouraging young people to participate in community action. The decline of the nuclear family, without any compensating community ties, bonds, and loyalties must somehow be ameliorated. Young people can only begin to see health and life as something to be taken seriously if they become imbued with a sense of purpose in the family, community, and workplace.[51]

Notes

1. National Safety Council, *Accident Facts, 1974* (National Safety Council, 1974), pp. 60–61. Unless indicated otherwise, all mortality and morbidity statistics in this appendix refer to ages 15–24.

2. U.S., Department of Justice, *Uniform Crime Reports for the United States, 1973* (Washington, D.C.: GPO, 1973), p. 8.

3. U.S., Department of Health, Education, and Welfare, *U.S. Vital Statistics, Annual 1973,* vol. 2: *Mortality,* part A, preprint, p. 10; National Center for Health Statistics, telephone communication, March 28, 1975.

4. National Safety Council, *Accident Facts.*

5. *Ibid.,* p. 54.

6. *Ibid.,* p. 61.

7. National Safety Council, *Traffic Accident Facts, 1974* (National Safety Council, 1974).

8. *Ibid.;* Edward C. Burks, *New York Times,* February 23, 1975.

9. *U.S. Vital Statistics, Annual 1973,* vol. 2, p. 10.

10. Enid Nemy, *New York Times,* April 16, 1973.

11. U.S., Department of Commerce, Bureau of the Census, *Statistical Abstract of the United States, 1974,* p. 150.

12. National Commission on the Causes and Prevention of Violence, Final Report, *To Establish Justice, To Insure Domestic Tranquility* (Washington, D.C.: GPO, 1969), p. 22. See also, Ted Morgan, "They Think I Can Kill Because I'm 14," *New York Times Magazine,* January 19, 1975.

13. Richard Block et al., "Homicide in Chicago, 1965–1970," *Journal of Research in Crime and Delinquency,* vol. 10, no. 1, January 1973. See also, Selwyn Raab, "Felony Murder Rose Here Sharply in '74," *New York Times,* March 23, 1975.

14. U.S. Department of Justice, p. 8.

15. National Commission on the Causes and Prevention of Violence, p. 24.

16. U.S. Department of Justice, p. 59.

17. *Ibid.,* p. 6.

18. A. Joan Klebba, *Mortality Trends for Homicide, by Age, Color, and Sex: United States, 1960–1972 (With Glances at the Statistical Profiles of the Victims during 1900–59 and 1973),* National Center for Health Statistics, Division of Vital Statistics, November 1974 (processed).

19. Arnold Barnett et al., *On Urban Homicide: A Statistical Analysis,* working paper, Massachusetts Institute of Technology, Operations Research Center, Cambridge, March, 1974. Published summary in *Technology Review,* July/August 1974, pp. 49–50.

20. Metropolitan Life, *Statistical Bulletin,* vol. 55, November 1974, p. 2.

21. National Commission on the Causes and Prevention of Violence, p. 184.

22. *Statistical Abstract of the United States, 1974,* p. 151.

23. Nancy Hicks, "Fight Over Gun Control Faces Test as Levi Favors Curb", *New York Times,* April 8, 1975, p. 16.

24. Martin S. Geisel et al., "Effectiveness of State and Local Regulation of Handguns: A Statistical Analysis" in *Duke Law Journal*, vol. no. 4, 1969. As of March 1975, Detective Sergeant Morrocco, Firearms Division, New Jersey State Police, stated that New Jersey still has one of the most comprehensive handgun regulations in the nation and the murder and assault rate in the state is two-thirds of the national rate. Detective Sergeant Morrocco, telephone communication, March 19, 1975. On April 1, 1975, a new Massachusetts gun statute subjected anyone in the state convicted of carrying firearms illegally to a mandatory one-year jail term. *New York Times*, May 4, 1975, p. 32.

25. Metropolitan Life, p. 2.

26. C. Henry Kempe et al., "The Battered-Child Syndrome," *Journal of the American Medical Association*, vol. 181, July 1962, pp. 17–24.

27. The two most rigorous analytical studies presently are David G. Gil, *Violence against Children: Physical Abuse in the United States* (Cambridge, Mass.: Harvard University Press, 1970); and Richard J. Light, "Abused and Neglected Children in America; A Study of Alternatives," *Harvard Educational Review*, vol. 43, no. 4, November 1973, pp. 556–98. See also, New Jersey Division of Youth and Family Services, *Abuse and Neglect in New Jersey; Estimating the Incidence per County, Projecting Treatment Needs, Descriptions of Treatment Programs*, August 1974, which estimated that during 1975, 25,000 children or 1.0 percent of all under 18, would be subjected to physical abuse or severe neglect.

28. Vincent Fontana, *The Maltreated Child: The Maltreatment Syndrome in Children*, 2d ed. (Springfield, Ill.: Charles C. Thomas, 1971).

29. Gil, *Violence against Children.*

30. *Ibid.*, p. 142.

31. Arthur Schlesinger, *Violence: America in the Sixties* (New York: Signet Books, 1968), p. 50.

32. National Commission on the Causes and Prevention of Violence, To Establish Justice, To Insure Domestic Tranquility, p. 199.

33. *Ibid.*, pp. 201–2.

34. Surgeon General's Scientific Advisory Committee on Television and Social Behavior, *Television and Growing Up: The Impact of Televised Violence*, U.S. Public Health Service, Washington, D.C., 1972, pp. 23–24.

35. *Ibid.*, pp. 17–18.

36. Linda Charlton, "Study Aides Voice Misgivings about Report on TV Violence," *New York Times*, February 19, 1972.

37. Surgeon General's Scientific Advisory Committee on Television and Social Behavior, *Television and Growing Up*, p. 33.

38. Eli A. Rubinstein, "The TV Violence Report: What's Next?" *Journal of Communication*, vol. 24, no. 1, Winter 1974, pp. 81–88.

39. U.S., Congress, Senate, Subcommittee on Communications of the Committee on Commerce, *Hearings on the Surgeon General's Report by the Scientific Advisory Committee on Television and Social Behavior*, 92d Cong., 2d sess., March 1972.

40. U.S., Congress, Senate, Subcommittee on Communications of the Committee on Commerce, *Hearings on Department of Health, Education, and Welfare's Progress in Developing a Profile on Violence on Television*, 93d Cong., 2d sess., April 1974, p. 1.

41. The proposed violence index is to be a development of Dr. George Gerbner's TV profile, which was an important source for both the Eisenhower Commission and the Surgeon General's committee. One month of prime TV time is taped each year at the Annenberg School of

Communications and coded for content by comprehensive indices. Dr. Eli Rubenstein, Vice-Chairman of the Surgeon General's Committee, telephone communication, March 28, 1975.

42. Federal Communications Commission, *Report on the Broadcast of Violent, Indecent, and Obscene Material*, February 19, 1975, p. 5.

43. *Ibid.*, Appendix B, p. 2.

44. *Ibid.*, p. 6.

45. Stanley Milgram et al., *Television and Antisocial Behavior: Field Experiments* (New York: Academic Press, 1973); Douglass Cater and Stephen Strickland, *TV Violence and the Child: The Surgeon General's Quest* (New York: Russel Sage, 1975); Alberta E. Siegel, "Televised Violence: Recent Research on Its Effects," in *Aggression: Proceedings of the Association for Research in Nervous and Mental Disease, December 1972* (Baltimore: Williams and Wilkins Co., 1974), pp. 271–283.

46. William Gale, "What Does a Street Gang Watch on the 'Trick Box'?" *New York Times*, March 30, 1975.

47. National Commission on the Causes and Prevention of Violence, *To Establish Justice, To Insure Domestic Tranquility*, p. xxi.

48. *Ibid.*, p. 20. However, the number of murder victims in proportion to population was highest in the Southern states, with 12.9 murders per 100,000 inhabitants in 1973. U.S., Department of Justice, *Uniform Crime Reports for the United States, 1973*, p. 6.

49. Tom Wicker, "Jobs and Crime," *New York Times*, May 4, 1975, p.33.

50. *Crimes of Violence*, A Staff Report to the National Commission of the Causes and Prevention of Violence, vol. 12 (1969), p. 667.

51. A. R. Somers, "Death Rates, Lifestyle, and National Morale: Two Proposals," *Bulletin of the American Protestant Hospital Association*, Spring 1972, pp. 4–29; A. R. Somers, "Adapting Institutions to Changing Needs," *Hospitals*, vol. 48, May 1, 1974, pp. 41–44.

Appendix H
Behavior Modification: A Review of Basic Concepts and Recent Research

by
Frederic Bass, M.D., D.Sc.*

BASIC CONCEPTS AND HISTORY

Behavior modification is relatively new; the field represents an extension of basic research on animal learning by I. P. Pavlov and B. F. Skinner to problems in human behavior.[1] The behavioral approach is characterized by an emphasis on relating measurable activity (responses) to antecedent and subsequent environmental events (stimuli).

Two of the concepts growing out of this approach—contingency management and stimulus control—have proved particularly productive. Contingency management is based on the experimental observation that consequences of behavior (reinforcing stimuli) determine the pattern of subsequent behavior; thus, a reinforcer is a behavioral consequence which has the effect of making the behavior which preceded it or produced it more likely to be repeated.[2] A reward, such as praise or money given for making a designated behavior, is an example of a reinforcer.

A second important concept is stimulus control, which analyzes how stimuli provide the context for on-going behavior.[3] A stimulus can affect behavior either because the stimulus has been associated with a reinforcer or because the stimulus signals a situation where the behavior has been associated with a reinforcer. Stimulus control analysis is used in many behavioral applications to determine exactly how the environment controls problem behavior; typically, a detailed record is made of current mood, physical location, social context, and the defining characteristics of each occurrence of maladaptive behavior.

*Department of Community Medicine, University of Pennsylvania School of Medicine, Philadelphia, Pennsylvania. This appendix is adapted from O. Pomerleau, Ph.D., F. Bass, M.D., D.Sc., and V. Crown, M.P.H., "The Role of Behavior Modification in Preventive Medicine," *New England Journal of Medicine* (forthcoming).

Behavioral concepts have been applied to human problems such as alcoholism,[4] mental retardation,[5] neurosis,[6] psychosis,[7] anorexia nervosa,[8] childhood autism,[9] chronic pain,[10] depression,[11] hysteria,[12] phobias,[13] poor study habits,[14] and stuttering.[15]

RECENT RESEARCH

The recent emergence of specialized behavioral techniques for enhancing "self-control" has important implications for the application of behavior modification to problems in preventive medicine.[16] In many of the examples cited above, change was brought about through environmental manipulations which modified the behavior of the person with the problem; in self-control procedures, however, the person with the problem modifies aspects of his environment which in turn modify the problem behavior. Thus, with self-control methods the passive role of patient is transformed into the active one of participant and therapist.

The behavioral treatment of obesity has a well-documented record of effectiveness. Of the early attempts to treat obesity by behavioral means, the work of C. B. Ferster, J. I. Nurnberger, and E. E. Levitt has been most influential.[17] Among the developments which grew out of their work were (a) a stimulus-control analysis based on written record of daily eating being overeating, (b) the specification and subsequent disruption of the reinforcers maintaining overeating, (c) the development of new reinforcers for behaviors which could serve as alternatives to overeating, and (d) the identification of the "ultimate aversive consequences" of overeating to provide a rationale and motivation for attempting behavior change. The approach is a direct application of operant reinforcement principles derived from the animal laboratory to the problem of overeating.

R. B. Stuart adapted Ferster's self-control approach to a small-group setting (to provide social reinforcement) and devised the following innovations: (a) a stimulus-control analysis based on a written record of daily eating behavior; (b) the reduction of total caloric intake by limiting the number of situations in which eating was authorized (e.g., eating in only one specified place in the home); (c) an assessment of progress in avoiding the ultimate aversive consequences by keeping track of weight on a weekly basis; and (d) the development of techniques to increase behavioral control (e.g., shopping for food after a meal rather than before, eating more slowly to allow time for satiation, etc.).[18]

In a series of formal, controlled comparisons, A. J. Stunkard and his co-workers replicated Stuart's findings and demonstrated that a behavioral approach to weight reduction was more effective than traditional approaches.[19] Behavioral methods have been used since then in various situations, for example, with obese schizophrenic patients,[20] overweight women in a general hospital,[21] self-help groups for the overweight,[22] etc.

Although the clinical management of obesity using behavioral methods is more advanced, a number of recent developments in the treatment of smoking and alcoholism suggest that a similar approach may be equally effective for these disorders.[23]

A recent study by A. J. Meyer and J. B. Henderson compared the effectiveness of behavior modification with other treatment methods in reducing the risk of cardiovascular disease in an industrial population.[24] Subjects were assigned to one of the following treatments: (a) twelve behavior-modification sessions using self-control techniques lasting two to three hours in a group setting, (b) nine 15-minute individual counseling sessions with a health educator, or (c) one 20-minute counseling session with a physician. Treatment lasted for eleven weeks and was followed by a post-treatment evaluation at the end of three months. For each group, the treatment goals were to decrease the consumption of saturated fats and carbohydrates, to lower overall caloric intake, to increase the level of physical activity, and to terminate or reduce the amount of cigarette smoking.

The results showed that behavior modification produced greater changes in health habits than the other procedures and that the improvements observed were more lasting. Individual counseling with a health educator was less effective than behavior modification, but was clearly superior to a single consultation with a physician. All three procedures resulted in improvements in the physiological measurements of risk—blood cholesterol and triglyceride levels.

The clinical research described above, taken as a whole, points toward the feasibility of a behavioral approach to preventive medicine. While the examples given in the present context have involved overeating, smoking, excessive alcohol consumption, and the prevention of cardiovascular disease, the techniques developed can be applied to any pattern of behavior which has medical implications. Thus, with suitable adjustment for clinical and situational differences, similar techniques could be used for improving personal health habits (for example, getting people to use dental floss regularly), improving patients' cooperation with physicians' recommendations (for example, by keeping clinic appointments), and increasing the effectiveness of medical treatment (for example, getting patients to take prescribed drugs in the early, asymptomatic stage of hypertension.)

Notes

1. I. P. Pavlov, *Conditioned Reflexes* (New York: Dover Publications, 1927); B. F. Skinner, *The Behavior of Organisms* (New York: Appleton-Century-Crofts, 1938).

2. B. F. Skinner, *Science and Human Behavior* (New York: MacMillan, 1953); H. Rachlin, *Introduction to Modern Behaviorism* (San Francisco: W. H. Freeman, 1970).

3. Skinner, *Science and Human Behavior;* H. Terrace, "Stimulus Control," in W. K. Honig, ed., *Operant Behavior: Areas of Research and Application* (New York: Appleton-Century-Crofts, 1966).

4. J. Thimann, "Conditioned Reflex Treatment of Alcoholism: Its Rationale and Technic,"*New England Journal of Medicine*, vol. 241, 1949, pp. 368–70; W. C. Voegtlin, "The Treatment of Alcoholism by Establishing a Conditioned Reflex," *American Journal of Medical Science*, vol. 199, 1940, pp. 802–09.

5. P. R. Fuller, "Operant Conditioning in a Vegetative Human Organism," *American Journal of Psychology*, vol. 62, 1949, pp. 587–90.

6. H. J. Eysenck, "The Effects of Psychotherapy: An Evaluation," *Journal of Consulting Psychology*, vol. 16, 1952, pp. 319–24; J. Wolpe, "Experimental Neurosis as Learned Behavior," *British Journal of Psychology*, vol. 43, 1952, p. 243.

7. O. R. Lindsley, "Operant Conditioning Methods Applied to Research in Chronic Schizophrenia," *Psychiatric Research Reports*, vol. 5, 1956, pp. 118–39; T. Ayllon and N. Azrin, *The Token Economy: A Motivational System for Therapy and Rehabilitation* (New York: Appleton-Century-Crofts, 1968).

8. A. Bachrach, W. Erwin, and J. Mohr, "The Control of Eating Behavior in an Anoretic by Operant Conditioning Techniques," in L. P. Ullman and L. Krasner, eds., *Case Studies in Behavior Modification* (New York: Holt, Rinehart and Winston, 1965); H. Leitenberg, W. Agras, and L. Thompson, "A Sequential Analysis of the Effect of Selective Positive Reinforcement in Modifying Anorexia Nervosa," *Behavior Research and Therapy*, vol. 6, 1968, pp. 211–18.

9. C. Ferster, "An Operant Reinforcement Analysis of Infantile Autism," in S. Lesse, ed., *An Evaluation of the Results of Psychotherapies* (Springfield, Ill.; Charles Thomas, 1968); I. Dovaas, B. Schaeffer, and J. Simmons, "Building Social Behavior in Autistic Children by Use of Electric Shock," *Journal of Experimental Research in Personality*, vol. 1, 1965, pp. 99–109.

10. W. Fordyce, R. Fowler, J. Lehmann, and B. DeLateur, "Some Implications of Learning in Problems of Chronic Pain," *Journal of Chronic Disease*, vol. 21, 1968, pp. 179–90; R. Fowler, W. Fordyce, and R. Berni, "Operant Conditioning in Chronic Illness," *American Journal of Nursing*, 1969, pp. 1226–28.

11. M. Hersen, R. Eisler, G. Alford, and W. Agras, "Effect of a Token Economy on Neurotic Depression: An Experimental Analysis," *Behavior Therapy*, vol. 4, 1973, pp. 392–97.

12. J. P. Brady and O. L. Lind, "Experimental Analysis of Hysterical Blindness," *Archives of General Psychiatry*, vol. 4, 1961, pp. 331–39; H. J. Grosz and J. Zimmerman, "Experimental Analysis of Hysterical Blindness: A Follow-up Report and New Experimental Data," *Archives of General Psychiatry*, vol. 13, 1965, p. 225–60.

13. J. Wolpe and A. Lazarus, *Behavior Therapy Techniques* (New York: Pergamon Press, 1966).

14. I. Goldiamond, "Self-Control Procedures in Personal Behavior Problems," *Psychological Reports*, vol. 17, 1965, pp. 851–58.

15. J. P. Brady, "Metronome-Conditioned Speech Retraining for Stuttering," *Behavior Therapy*, vol. 2, 1971, pp. 129–50.

16. M. R. Goldfried and M. Merbaum, *Behavior Change through Self-Control* (New York: Holt, Rinehart and Winston, 1973); M. Mahoney and C. Thoreson, *Self-Control: Power to the Person* (Monterey, Cal.: Brooks/Cole, 1974).

17. C. B. Ferster, J. I. Nurnberger, and E. E. Levitt, "The Control of Eating," *Journal of Mathetics*, vol. 1, 1962, pp. 87–109.

18. R. B. Stuart, "Behavioral Control of Overeating," *Behavior Research and Therapy*, vol. 5, 1967, pp. 357–65; R. B. Stuart and B. Davis, *Slim Chance in a Fat World: Behavioral Control*

of Obesity (Champaign, Ill.: Research Press, 1971).

19. S. B. Penick, R. Filion, S. Fok, and A. J. Stunkard, "Behavior Modification in the Treatment of Obesity," *Psychosomatic Medicine*, vol. 33, 1971, pp. 49–55; A. J. Stunkard, "New Therapies for the Eating Disorders," *Archives of General Psychiatry*, vol. 26, 1972, pp. 391–98.

20. M. Harmatz and P. Lapuc, "Behavior Modification of Overeating in a Psychiatric Population," *Journal of Consulting and Clinical Psychology*, vol. 32, 1968, pp. 583–87.

21. W. Shipman, "Behavior Therapy with Obese Dieters," *Annual Report of the Institute for Psychosomatic and Psychiatric Research and Training* (Michael Reese Medical Center, 1970), pp. 70–71.

22. L. Levita and A. J. Stunkard, "A Therapeutic Coalition for Obesity: Behavior-Modification and Patient Self-Help," *American Journal of Psychiatry*, vol. 131, 1974, pp. 423–27.

23. J. Tooley and S. Pratt, "An Experimental Procedure for the Extinction of Smoking Behavior," *Psychological Record*, vol. 17, 1967, pp. 209–18; O. F. Pomerleau and P. Ciccone, "Preliminary Results of a Treatment Program for Smoking Cessation Using Multiple Behavior Modification Techniques," paper presented to the annual meeting of the American Association for Behavior Therapy, Chicago, 1974; D. Ober, "The Modification of Smoking Behavior," *Journal of Consulting and Clinical Psychology*, vol. 32, 1968, pp. 543–49; F. Cheek, C. Franks, J. Laucius, and V. Burtle, "Behavior Modification Training for Wives of Alcoholics," *Quarterly Journal of Studies on Alcohol*, vol. 32, 1971, pp. 456–61; G. Hunt and N. Azrin, "A Community-Reinforcement Approach to Alcoholism," *Behavior Research and Therapy*, vol. 11, 1973, pp. 91–104; L. Sobel and M. Sobel, "A Self-Feedback Technique to Monitor Drinking Behavior in Alcoholics," *Behavior Research and Therapy*, vol. 11, 1973, pp. 237–38; C. Holden, "Alcoholism: On the Job Referrals Mean Early Detection, Treatment," *Science*, vol. 179, 1973, p. 363; P. Miller, "The Use of Behavioral Contracting in the Treatment of Alcoholism: A Case Report," *Behavior Therapy*, vol. 3, 1972, pp. 593–96; J. Ray, "Drug Abuse in Business: Part of a Larger Problem," *Personnel*, vol. 49, 1972, pp. 1-3; M. Cohen, I. Liebson, L. Faillace, and W. Speers, "Alcoholism: Controlled Drinking and Incentive for Abstinence," *Psychological Reports*, vol. 28, 1971, pp. 575–80; J. Ewing and B. Rouse, "Outpatient Group Treatment to Inculcate Controlled Drinking Behavior in Alcoholics," paper presented to the International Congress on Alcoholism and Drug Dependence, Amsterdam, 1972; F. Gottheil, B. Murphy, T. Skoloda, and L. Corbett, "Fixed Interval Drinking II: Drinking and Discomfort in 25 Alcoholics," *Quarterly Journal of Studies on Alcohol*, vol. 33, 1972, pp. 325–40; P. Miller and D. Barlow, "Behavioral Approaches to the Treatment of Alcoholism," *Journal of Nervous and Mental Disease*, vol. 157, 1973, pp. 10–20; H. Schaefer, "Twelve-Month Follow-up of Behaviorally Trained Ex-Alcoholic Social Drinkers," *Behavior Therapy*, vol. 3, 1972, pp. 286–89; M. B. Sobell and L. C. Sobell, *Individualized Behavior Therapy for Alcoholics*, Research Monograph no. 13 (State of California Department of Mental Hygiene, 1972).

24. A. J. Meyer and J. B. Henderson, "Multiple Risk Factor Reduction in the Prevention of Cardiovascular Disease," *Preventive Medicine*, vol. 3, 1974, pp. 225–336.

Appendix I
Report from Committee on Health
Education
to
Health Insurance Benefits Advisory
Council
Transmitted to
the Secretary of Health, Education,
and Welfare
February 15, 1974
from
Annual Report of
the Health Insurance Benefits
Advisory Council
July 1, 1973 — June 30, 1974

HEALTH INSURANCE BENEFITS ADVISORY COUNCIL

Honorable Caspar W. Weinberger
Secretary of Health, Education,
and Welfare
330 Independence Avenue, SW
Washington, D.C. 20201

Dear Mr. Secretary:

The Health Insurance Benefits Advisory Council, through its Committee
on Health Education, has been studying the issue of consumer health
education and has adopted the enclosed report developed by the
Committee.

To summarize briefly, the Council supports defining health education
as a professional discipline, and development of a national policy on
health education. It also would encourage Medicare reimbursement for
preventive health education programs, with particular emphasis on
utilizing the experimental provisions of P.L. 92-603. To the extent
consonant with the law, the report also reflects the Council's feeling
that Medicare reimbursement should be consistent with the provision
in P.L. 93-222 requiring that an HMO, in order to obtain Federal
start-up funds, must provide health education services. The Council
recommended broad dissemination of information on the present coverage
for health education activities provided under Medicare, Medicaid and
the Maternal and Child Health and Crippled Children's Programs.

The Council has also gone on record in general support of the
recommendation of the President's Committee on Health Education for
establishment of a National Center for Health Education and, in
clarification of the Committee's generalized recommendation for a
"focal point" within the Department, recommends a high-level Office of
Consumer Health Education be established in DHEW to coordinate and
upgrade existing health education programs.

The Committee will continue its activities and the Council is prepared
to cooperate with the Department as health education policies develop.

Sincerely yours,

Ernest W. Baward, M.D.
Acting Chairman
Health Insurance Benefits
Advisory Council

Enclosure

REPORT FROM THE COMMITTEE ON HEALTH EDUCATION
to
HEALTH INSURANCE BENEFITS ADVISORY COUNCIL
January 11, 1974

Introduction: The Importance of Defining and Implementing
              National Policy for Health Education

Consumer health education is an idea whose time has come. This
fact is increasingly accepted by consumers and providers, by educators
and third-party payers, by leaders of both public and private sectors.

Underlying this development is the growing recognition that
individual lifestyle and individual behavior are major risk-factors
influencing the mortality and morbidity of the American people. Heart
disease and accidents - two of our four major killers - can usually
be traced to lifestyle . In the case of stroke, life style is an
important contributing factor. It is probably primary in the case of
emphysema, cirrhosis, and at least two cancers.

It is the primary factor in venereal disease and primary or
contributory with respect to most chronic illness, including obesity,
alcoholism, drug abuse and the other addictions, most mental illness,
high blood pressure, ulcer, and diabetes.

Even where the primary causal factor of illness is due to heredity,
environmental pollution, or some other cause beyond control of the
individual, his ability to cope and to lead a reasonably normal life
depends on his lifestyle.

The good physician and the good nurse have always recognized the
importance of patient education as an integral part of patient care.
In recent years, more and more hospitals and community health centers
have developed organized patient education programs as part of routine
patient care and discharge procedures. Even more recently, some
have extended these programs to include outreach to non-patients
living in the hospital's community or service area, especially those
with addictions and other high-risk factors for coronary and other
diseases.

Despite these efforts on the part of individual health professionals
and institutions, it is widely believed that a far greater emphasis
is needed - both on education of individual patients and of the
community at large. Appointment of the President's Committee on Health
Education and the release of its Report in October 1973 are evidence
of the growing national commitment of health education.

HIBAC welcomes this Report and acknowledges with appreciation its contribution to definition and development of national policy in this long-neglected area.

HIBAC also notes with approval the demonstration project in hospital-based consumer health education currently being conducted by the College of Medicine and Dentistry of New Jersey - Rutgers Medical School as reported to this Council November 16, 1973.

However, it is clear that health education, as a professional discipline, is still inadequately defined and developed. This is not surprising in view of the fact that the objectives of health education and its relation to the health professions in general are also inadequately defined. If health education is to achieve its potential and accomplish the goals of the President's Committee and the CMDNJ-RMS demonstration project, it must establish itself as an effective component of the health care team with defined goals, and criteria and methodology for evaluation of progress toward these goals. It is too late in the day for the advocates of health education to try to "sell" themselves simply as another well-meaning effort to solve the U.S. "health care crisis."

In the words of the CMDNJ-RMS statement presented to this Council,

"The value of any health education program - whether a multi-million dollar national program or a single project costing a few hundred dollars - must ultimately be judged not on the basis of the size of its budget, the number of classes held, pieces of literature distributed or other input data, but in terms of actual consumer behavior modification and outcome as measured by objective indices of health."

The general thrust of a national health education policy, at this time, should be along two complementary lines:

1.   Encouragement - by means of financial, technical, informational, political, moral, and other assistance - of new programs and demonstration projects, involving both patient education and general public education, especially in settings where meaningful evaluation can be carried out; and

2.   By the same means - encouragement of and, as a condition of general program support, insistence on training, evaluation, and other activities designed to improve the quality and quantity of personnel available for health education and the quality of programs being offered.

In all respects - program development, personnel training, and evaluation - special emphasis must be placed on behavior modification.

Recommendations

In accordance with our instructions from Dr. Saward, Acting Chairman of HIBAC, on November 16, 1973, the Committee on Health Education addressed itself to two specific issues:

1. Criteria for reimbursement by Medicare and Medicaid of hospital-based patient education; and

2. Implementation of the major recommendations of the President's Committee.

Reimbursement

We have noted with approval the recommendation of the President's Committee:

"That the government, prepayment plans and insurance companies, which pay for health care services to others, be willing to adjust premium rates to include in their payments the cost of health education to the patients involved" (Report, p. 25).

We strongly urge the private carriers to implement this recommendation as rapidly as possible.

We have noted with approval the provision of the new HMO Act of 1973 making health education a requirement for Federal funding.

We have also consulted with the staff of the School Security Administration and the Medical Services Administration and have received the attached letters from Mr. Tierney, Director, Bureau of Health Insurance, Social Security Administration, and Mr. Newman, Commissioner, Medical Services Administration, Social and Rehabilitation Service.

With respect to Medicare, the principal points set forth in Mr. Tierney's letter may be summarized as follows:

1. Institutional and home care patient education programs which are an integral part of the treatment of illness and injury are reimbursable under Medicare;

2. Programs which are purely preventive are not generally reimbursable;

3. Selected programs which meet the requirements of P.L. 92-603 for experiments in reimbursement may be funded by SSA on an experimental basis even though they may involve prevention.

The Committee believes it would also be desirable for Medicare
to reimburse for health education programs designed to prevent illness
and injury and hence the need for expensive medical and hospital services.
Such reimbursement is essential to be consistent with the new HMO law
and we believe that the Medicare law will require amendment along these
lines. However, we recognize the constraints of the present law and,
within these constraints, the three points set forth above seem to
us to provide a sensible present basis for Medicare reimbursement. In
particular, we are pleased that Point 3 permits the advocates of health
education to apply for grants to conduct additional pilot experiments
and to demonstrate health education's potential for greater cost
effectiveness.

With respect to Medicaid, in addition to reimbursement for
institutional and home care educational programs, there are three other
possibilities as indicated in Mr. Newman's letter: for recipients who
receive their care through HMOs, through OEO neighborhood health centers
that are reimbursed on the basis of an all-inclusive rate, or for children
reached through the Early & Periodic Screening and Diagnosis Program.
In the latter case, the Federal guidelines actively encourage related
educational programs. Reimbursement is also encouraged under title V,
Maternal and Child Health and Crippled Children's Programs.

RECOMMENDATION 1. THAT HIBAC RECOMMEND TO THE SECRETARY OF
H.E.W. THAT INFORMATIONAL MATERIALS INCORPORATING THE ABOVE POINTS
BE FORMULATED AND MADE AVAILABLE, AS SOON AS POSSIBLE, TO ALL
APPROPRIATE PROVIDERS AND THIRD-PARTY INTERMEDIARIES AND CARRIERS.

RECOMMENDATION 2. THAT ALL APPROPRIATE GOVERNMENTAL HEALTH
AND INSURANCE DEPARTMENTS AND AGENCIES, UNIONS AND OTHER CONSUMER
REPRESENTATIVES BE INFORMED OF THESE POSSIBILITIES FOR FEDERAL THIRD-
PARTY REIMBURSEMENT AND GRANTS SO THAT CONSUMERS MAY BE ALERTED TO THESE
SERVICES AND THEIR ENTITLEMENT THERETO.

President's Committee

We agree with the President's Committee on the need for two
specific actions to give immediate visibility and support to health
education:

1.   Establishment of a new quasi-public National Center for
Health Education to be chartered by the Congress but supported by a
combination of public and private funds and under the policy
direction of a Board representing both the public and private sectors
(Report, pp. 22, 28-31).

2.   Establishment of a "focal point" within the Department of
H.E.W. "to help make the Federal Government's involvement in health
education more effective and more efficient" (Report, p. 24).

We <u>do not</u> support every aspect of the Committee's recommendations with respect to organization of the National Center. We <u>do</u> believe that the concept of a "focal point" needs clarification, probably involving creation of a high-level Office of Consumer Health Education within H.E.W. to be responsible for coordinating and upgrading most of the existing health education programs now scattered throughout the Department.

In general, however, we believe that these two actions - coupled with more clearly defined reimbursement policies – could go a long way toward helping to establish an effective national health education policy.

RECOMMENDATION 3.   THAT HIBAC RECOMMEND TO THE SECRETARY OF H.E.W. ESTABLISHMENT, AS SOON AS POSSIBLE, OF A HIGH-LEVEL OFFICE OF CONSUMER HEALTH EDUCATION.

RECOMMENDATION 4.   THAT HIBAC RECOMMEND TO THE SECRETARY OF H.E.W. FORMULATION AND SUBMISSION TO THE CONGRESS, AS SOON AS POSSIBLE, OF LEGISLATION AUTHORIZING ESTABLISHMENT OF A NATIONAL CENTER FOR HEALTH EDUCATION WITH SUPPORTING FUNDS ALONG THE GENERAL LINES RECOMMENDED BY THE PRESIDENT'S COMMITTEE ON HEALTH EDUCATION.

Respectfully submitted,

Anne R. Somers, Chairman
Melnea A. Cass
J. Rodney Feild, M.D.
Sam A. McConnell, Jr.

Attachments: 2

DEPARTMENT OF HEALTH, EDUCATION, AND WELFARE

Mrs. Anne Somers, Director
Office of Consumer Health Education
College of Medicine and Dentistry
of New Jersey--Rutgers Medical School
Piscataway, New Jersey 08854

Dear Anne:

This is the statement of our policy we prepared in accordance with your
recent discussion with Bob Hoyer concerning Medicare reimbursement for
hospital-based consumer health education programs.

While the Medicare law does not specifically identify patient education
programs as covered hospital services, our policy is that reimbursement
may be made under the program to the extent that the programs are
appropriate parts in the rendition of covered services. Covered services
must be reasonable and necessary to the treatment of the individual's
illness or injury. Working within this framework the program has helped
pay the costs of various types of educational activities. For example,
under the renal disease provision of the 1972 amendments, reimbursement is
made for training necessary to enable patients to dialyze at home.
Similarly, educational activities carried out by nurses--teaching patients
to give themselves injections, follow prescribed diets, administer
colostomy care, administer medical gases and carry out other patient care
activities--are reimbursable as part of covered nursing care. Similarly,
the instruction of a patient in the carrying out of a maintenance program
designed for him by a physical therapist is reimbursed as a part of
covered physical therapy.

Where, however, the educational activities are not closely related to the
care and treatment of the patient, such as programs directed toward
instructing patients or the public generally in preventive health care
activities, reimbursement cannot be made since the law limits payment
under the program to covered care which is reasonable and necessary to the
treatment of an illness or injury. For example, programs designed to
prevent illness by instructing the general public in the importance of
good nutritional habits, exercise regimens, and good hygiene are not
reimbursable under the program. I'm sure that no measures are taken,
however, to identify and eliminate the cost of an occasional lecture for
the benefit of patients, staff, and public on general health matters.

It seems to me there may be some advantage in considering this proposal under the experimentation provisions of Public Law 92-603, which authorizes the Secretary to make payments for services not now covered under either Medicare or Medicaid. If you agree, I recommend that you get in touch with Mr. Ronald H. Carlson, the Director of the Division of Special Operations, which has responsibility for our program experimentation activities in the Bureau. I have already sent him a copy of the material, so he will be familiar with the matter in the event you should call him. He can be reached at area code 301, 594-8000.

Sincerely yours,

Thomas M. Tierney
Director
Bureau of Health Insurance

DEPARTMENT OF HEALTH, EDUCATION, AND WELFARE

Mrs. Anne Somers, Director
Office of Consumer Health Education
College of Medicine and Dentistry
 of New Jersey
Rutgers Medical School
Piscataway, New Jersey 08854

Dear Anne:

I read with interest the subcommittee report on consumer health
education and certainly agree that it is an idea whose time has
come.

As you know, Medicaid reimbursement can and does cover educational
and preventive services provided to recipients who elect to
obtain their health care from a prepaid group practice plan such
as G.H.A. as well as other HMOs. Additionally, Medicaid has
reimbursed through the all-inclusive rate mechanism, for such
items of care provided by OEO neighborhood health centers,
community health centers, maternal and child health clinics,
etc. unless the single State agency administering the title XIX
program elects to pay for only the specified services covered
under the State Medicaid plan.

There is one other area of reimbursement for patient education
services to which I should like to call your attention. There
is a strong concentration on preventive services throughout
the early and periodic screening, diagnosis, and treatment
program, a basic service under title XIX. The provision of
services under this program should impart to the elegible
Medicaid patient the value of preventive and early detection
measures, e.g. immunizations. Reimbursement for services under
EPSDT is matched under title XIX at the medical assistance rate.
In addition guidelines for administration of the program which
have been distributed to the States encourage State agencies to
"actively seek out individuals for the EPSDT program" and "to
make sure that they understand the nature and purpose of the
screening program."

Page 2 - Mrs. Anne Somers, Director

The guidelines further specify a variety of information methods
designed to educate recipients about the availability of EPSDT
services. In part, the guidelines state:

> Some families will need help: (1) in understanding
> the importance of preventive health services and early
> diagnosis and treatment, (2) in overcoming their fears
> of doctors and other aspects of medical care, (3) in
> mobilizing themselves to make use of a health service
> for which they may feel no pressing need, and (4) in
> arranging for transportation, babysitting services or
> other services to enable parents to bring children to
> the screening center or to other providers of health
> services. Parents who are burdened with other family
> problems and financial stress may not be able to make
> much effort to seek screening examinations for their
> seemingly well children.

Services of this nature would be reimbursable under title XIX,
or as a social service under title IV-A of the Social Security
Act.

I trust this information will be useful to you and your committee.

Sincerely yours,

Howard N. Newman
Commissioner

Appendix J
Blue Cross Association
White Paper:
Patient Health Education

This White Paper addresses the issue of patient health education and the operational role which Blue Cross Plans can assume in this area. It finds that a patient education program, integrated into the routine services of the institution, offers the potential for both cost containment and improved quality of patient care. It concludes with the recommendation that Blue Cross Plans should encourage health care institutions to establish and operate programs in patient education and should support them financially through the existing payment mechanism. Approved by Blue Cross Association, Board of Governors, August 1974

The health care system is being challenged to improve its efficiency and effectiveness. Reforms in the system must forcefully address the need to contain rising health care costs and to assure the quality of health care services.

Given the complexity and the diversity of this challenge, no single response is appropriate. As one mechanism among many, patient health education may contribute to containing health care costs and enhancing the individual's understanding of and compliance with his treatment regimen. Patient education reinforces the patient's awareness of his responsibility for his own health, and self-responsibility is crucial for the ultimate effectiveness of health care.

Patient health education, for the present purpose, is a process comprising several elements: mutual identification of present and future health care needs by patient and professional, planning for the appropriate mix of professional and patient responsibility for meeting those needs, exchange of knowledge regarding the selected treatment regimen, motivation of patient and professional to perform their respective roles, and continuing evaluation of alternative methodologies. Patient education is part of the total process of patient care. As used here, patient education generally refers to hospital-based programs. However, the locus of the intervention is not as important as its nature.

The purpose of this statement is twofold: to examine the evidence on the impact of patient health education on the cost and quality of patient care and to recommend an operational course of action to Plans.

145

ISSUES

The concept of patient health education raises several issues. The principal questions which must be resolved, however, are:

1. Should Plans pay for patient education?
2. What kinds of criteria should be employed to determine the allocatability of patient education expenses to Plan reimbursement?
3. What is the appropriate role for Plans in patient health education?

The answers to such questions emerge from an evaluation of the impact of patient education on the cost and quality of health care.

Effects on Costs

In examining the costs of patient care, one may adopt several perspectives: health care costs per capita in a given service area, costs per admission, costs per service unit, and costs per episode of illness. The development of valid and reliable measures is crucial to the proper evaluation of the patient education program.

Theoretically, patient education might contribute to reduced costs by decreasing the unnecessary utilization of health care services and by encouraging use of the most appropriate locus of care for health problems. These potential effects are critical to improving the efficacy of medical services.

Empirical evidence suggests that structured patient education speeds recovery in certain case types. For example, preoperative instruction has resulted in a significantly higher incidence of early discharge among those receiving intensive preoperative instruction and practice as compared to those not receiving such treatment.[1] Other studies have found similar results. Specific educational interventions can lead to reduced use of postoperative narcotics,[2] decreased emergency room utilization,[3] decreased readmissions and patient days for readmissions,[4] and reduced total admissions for a target population.[5]

Total health care cost for the individual may be reduced by substituting less expensive treatment modalities and loci of care for hospitalization and emergency room use. To assess whether such substitutions really do reduce *total* costs, total utilization of health services by specific groups over a given time frame must be calculated.

While not presenting conclusive evidence of reduced *total* costs of care for specific groups, some studies do suggest large cost savings as a result of changes in the pattern of utilization. For example, the Tufts–New England Medical Center research, using a self-selected sample of male hemophiliac outpatients given postperiod instruction and practice in self-infusion, yielded the following pre-post comparisons: total inpatient days declined from 432 to 42, outpatient visits per patient decreased from 23.0 to 5.5, and total costs per patient went down 45 percent (from $5,780 to $3,209).[6] At the University of Southern California Medical Center, a reorganization of the diabetic care system, incorporating a telephone "hot line" for information, medical advice, and the filling of prescriptions, counseling by physicians and nurses, and pamphlets and posters to promote the service, was associated with more than a 50 percent reduction in emergency room visits per clinic patient and the avoidance of approximately 2,300 medication visits.[7] These findings suggest that certain types of patient education do promote the substitution of self-care and information-seeking for acute care services.

On balance, organized patient education has demonstrated its effectiveness in reducing the unnecessary utilization of certain health care services and in encouraging the use of the most appropriate, least-cost settings for care.

Effects on quality of care

Patient health education has also demonstrated considerable potential for improving the quality of care.

Several studies have demonstrated the beneficial impact of patient education on the *process* of patient care. The use of an interdisciplinary team to provide educationally oriented support to patients with congestive heart failure has resulted in increased knowledge among study patients in one sample regarding diet, medications, disease process, and, even more importantly, increased adherence to the treatment regimen.[8] Other research suggests that patient education enhances patient understanding of and compliance with the process of care.[9]

With respect to health care *outcomes*, studies have shown the quality-increasing effects of patient education. At the University of Southern California Medical Center, the reorganization of the system of diabetic care and the initiation of a multifaceted program of patient education was associated with a reduction of approximately two-thirds in the incidence of diabetic coma from 1968 to 1970.[10] Similarly, in another study, a significantly higher percentage of congestive heart failure patients receiving educational support improved in their ability to function, as measured by the American Heart Association classification. Also, recent work[11] at Massachusetts General Hospital has shown that the provision of intensive preoperative and postoperative information and guidance contributed to reduced pain among surgery patients. These studies point to the potential of patient education in enhancing health status.

CONCLUSION

The available information regarding patient health education indicates that, where conducted by a coordinated mix of educational and clinical specialists and directed to individual needs and capabilities, it both increases the quality of health care and presents potential cost savings to the health care system and to the public it serves. The Blue Cross system has consistently supported delivery and financing innovations which improve the systems's efficiency and effectiveness. As such, patient health education efforts should be encouraged and supported, for they are one promising means of achieving these objectives.

Accordingly, Plans should encourage health care institutions to establish and operate programs in patient education and should support them financially through the existing payment mechanism. To realize its full potential for cost savings and quality improvement, it is critical that the patient education function be integrated into the total process of patient care. To assure that sound programs are developed and maintained, the following guidelines are suggested as criteria for determining payment for patient education programs. In applying these guidelines, the variation in programs and population needs for patient education should be considered. Accordingly, a flexible approach to their interpretation should be adopted.

GUIDELINES FOR PROGRAMS IN PATIENT EDUCATION

1. The purpose and operational objectives of the program should be clearly stated, and the techniques for meeting the objectives should be specified.

2. Patient education should be provided as an integral element of the total patient care process within a supportive organizational framework.[12] Existing hospital-based programs in patient education shall be reviewed by either the Joint Commission on Accreditation of Hopitals or the Bureau of Hospitals of the American Osteopathic Association.

3. Necessary and appropriate health education should be developed and financed as a routine element of the care of each patient.

4. Educational methodologies should be directed to specific case types and desired behavioral changes and the results of such interventions as to cost and quality of care should be documented. As in other expenses, continuing management evaluation of the cost-effectiveness of the service should be conducted. Programs should be revised over time to reflect the results of such evaluation.

It is appropriate that the Blue Cross system encourage the development of cost-effective programs in patient education. Where patient education is properly related to the other components of the total patient care process, there is clear potential for reduction of health care costs and improvement in the quality of health care processes and outcomes. Blue Cross Plans share responsibility with those providing patient education to ensure that this potential is realized. Accordingly, the Blue Cross System should play an active part in the development, implementation, and evaluation of sound programs in patient education.

NOTES

1. Kathryn M. Healy, "Does Preoperative Instruction Really Make a Difference?" *American Journal of Nursing*, January 1968, pp. 62–67.

2. Lawrence D. Egbert et al., "Reduction of Postoperative Pain by Encouragement and Instruction of Patients," *New England Journal of Medicine*, April 16, 1974, pp. 825–27.

3. Leona Miller and Jack Goldstein, "More Efficient Care of Diabetic Patients in a County Hospital Setting," *New England Journal of Medicine*, June 29, 1972, pp. 1388–91.

4. Stanley G. Rosenberg, "Patient Education Leads to Better Care for Heart Patients," *Health Services Reports*, September 1971, pp. 793–802.

5. Ibid.

6. Peter H. Levine and Anthony F. Britten, "Supervised Patient Management of Hemophilia," *Annals of Internal Medicine*, no. 78, 1973, pp. 195-201.

7. See Miller and Goldstein, "More Efficient Care of Diabetic Patients."

8. Stanley G. Rosenberg, "Patient Education Leads to Better Care for Heart Patients."

9. Reported in Lawrence W. Green, "Toward Cost-Benefit Evaluations of Health Education: Some Concepts, Methods, and Examples," *Health Education Monographs*, vol. 2, supp. 1, May 1974, pp. 36–37.

10. Miller and Goldstein, "More Efficient Care of Diabetic Patients."

11. Egbert et al., "Reduction of Postoperative Pain."

12. Examples of this organizational framework are the hospital, home care, HMO, or community health education program.

Appendix K
A Public Health Approach to Unhealthy Behavior: The Example of Tuberculosis Control Applied to Cigarette Smoking

by
Frederic Bass, M.D., D. Sc.*

INTRODUCTION

With the growth of scientific knowledge in clinical technique in the modification of behavior, there is need for a framework with which to apply this knowledge systematically at the population level as well as clinically.[1] By organizing preventive care for the community as well as for the individual, successes will be obtained that would not otherwise be possible. The epidemiology of such problems, the organization of services, and the evaluation of the effectiveness of these services require consideration of the group in toto. The public health, disease control model, as it has been applied to tuberculosis, illustrates a coherent and well-organized community-level approach to prevention, and cigarette smoking represents one of the clearest, most serious and most readily identifiable behavioral risk factors to which such an approach might be translated.

THE PARADIGM OF TUBERCULOSIS CONTROL

The necessary conditions for success in approaching any disease or health problem affecting a population include:

1. The epidemiology of the condition is known. Epidemiology here means knowledge of the prevalence, incidence, natural history, risk factors, and transmission of the condition.

2. The condition is clearly identifiable and is routinely reported.

3. Diagnostic standards exist which have prognostic and therapeutic significance.

4. Methods of prevention have been evaluated and effective approaches defined.

5. Methods of treatment have been evaluated and the most effective

*Department of Community Medicine, University of Pennsylvania School of Medicine, Philadelphia, Pennsylvania; Member of Task Force on Consumer Health Education.

defined.

6. A role for the general medical care system with respect to the diagnosis and treatment of the problem has been defined and accepted by at least a significant minority of medical practitioners.

7. Social and psychological factors relating to diagnosis and treatment have been explored.

8. Society has assumed responsibility for controlling the condition.

9. Appropriate professional and public decision-making bodies have indentified target levels for the future prevalence of the condition.

10. Ethical and legal issues concerning societal authority versus individual rights have been recognized and considered.

1. Known Epidemiology

Over the past century the epidemiology of tuberculosis has been well elucidated. In fact, Koch's Postulates about tuberculosis epitomize the epidemiology of infectious disease.[2] The incidence of tuberculosis has been recorded in many nations. Its natural history has been described for humans, and its pathogenesis also observed in the laboratory.[3] Risk factors for the disease have been clearly identified. Its mode of spread has been ascertained on both an observational and experimental basis. And, it has been the subject of mathematical modeling to analyze the spread of the disease and the opportunities for its control.

2. Regularly Reported

Tuberculosis is a disease whose incidence has been reliably and broadly ascertained. Tuberculosis is one of the first chronic diseases whose treatment and follow-up have been systematically ascertained for the entire population. The tuberculosis-case register allows an assessment at any one point in time of how diagnosis and treatment stand for all reported cases.[4]

3. Diagnostic Standards

Diagnostic standards for tuberculosis have been formulated and revised according to the evolution of the clinical and epidemiological meanings of each diagnostic category.[5] Thus, anyone can be classified by whether he or she has had a reported case of tuberculosis, by whether the person has been a tuberculin reactor or not, by the person's last chest x-ray result, and by whether the person has had known exposure to a contagious case. Such an epidemiological classification provides tangible implications for diagnosis, therapy, and prevention.[6]

4. Prevention Rigorously Evaluated

The Medical Research Council of Great Britain and the U.S. Public Health Service have performed large-scale, controlled studies of various modes of prevention of tuberculosis. The efficacy of various vaccines against tuberculosis has been assessed in different populations.[7] After the development of Isoniazid, the value of chemoprophylaxis (i.e., the long-term administration of the drug to prevent the appearance of tuberculosis) was tested in various subgroups of the general population, subgroups categorized by tuberculin reactivity, chest x-ray result, and exposure to infectious cases of tuberculosis; the specific yield of chemoprophylaxis applied to various risk groups has been learned and articulated.[8]

5. Treatment Rigorously Evaluated

A number of dimensions of the treatment of tuberculosis have been tested through randomized controlled trials. The drugs given (their dosage, the duration for which they are prescribed, and whether they are given at one time during the day or in divided doses) and supplementary measures (bed rest, sanitorium vs. outpatient care, etc.) have been methodically evaluated.[9] Thus, because research has subjected all the principal variables of treatment to scrutiny, the physician treating tuberculosis today knows the potential use and value of each part of his armamentarium.

6. Social And Psychological Factors

A number of social and psychological variables have been examined, ranging from those concerned with diagnosis and treatment to those related to disease causation and rehabilitation. For example, patients' attitudes and behavior with respect to seeking care and obtaining checkups have been assessed and the results used in the planning and delivery of care.[10]

7. Societal Responsibility

One hundred years ago, Sir William Osler said that tuberculosis was a social problem with medical implications. In the intervening century, the public domain gradually has assumed full responsibility for the care of this condition. Money, personnel, services, and materials are now provided to diagnose, treat, and prevent tuberculosis as part of the protection of the entire community. Because of its epidemic potential, provision of care for all persons with tuberculosis or at risk of tuberculosis has protected and enhanced the well-being of all members of the community.

8. Defined Targets For The System

Tuberculosis has been one of the few health problems on which experts have conferred and set goals for future disease incidence, for levels of effectiveness in diagnosis and treatment, and for the extent of preventive care to be provided. Methods derived from scientific studies have formed the basis of these goals. The observed yields of various disease-control activities enabled prioritization of tasks and permitted a benefit-cost analysis of alternatives.[11]

Panels of experts appointed by the American Thoracic Society, after review of studies and after debate, have formulated specific criteria for diagnostic, preventive, and therapeutic measures. For example, 75 percent of newly-reported, active cases of tuberculosis should be culture-negative within three months of beginning drug therapy and 95 percent culture-negative within six months.[12] With the use of the tuberculosis case register, and now, with the use of the tuberculosis contact register, the status of treatment and prevention across an entire population can be assessed by those public health officials responsible for the care.

9. Ethical And Legal Issues

With the responsibility and authority given to public officials for controlling tuberculosis, an inevitable clash arose between the welfare of the general community and the individual's right to do as he pleased. As science defined more precisely the efficacy of drug treatment and the degree of infectiousness of various categories of patients, the ethical and legal basis for holding patients against their will diminished.[13] With the development of effective ambulatory care, the tuberculosis hospitals had lower and lower bed occupancy rates, and the authoritarian control that physicians maintained over the freedom of movement of their hospitalized patients subsided appropriately. Today, if the patient is hospitalized at all, the length of stay is a matter of weeks, whereas two decades ago it had been a matter of years.[14]

10. Relation To Conventional Medical Care

The hospitalization of tuberculosis patients in recent years has become the responsibility of the short-stay hospital.[15] The ambulatory care of the patient receiving chemotherapy is a responsibility of the primary care physician rather than the tuberculosis specialist. Furthermore, because of well-defined methods of diagnosis, prevention, and treatment, much of what needs to be done for tuberculosis patients has been delegated to nurses and to physician assistants; in effect, tuberculosis control has handed to general primary care a neatly packaged program.

THE TUBERCULOSIS PARADIGM APPLIED TO CIGARETTE SMOKING

1. Known Epidemiology

The initiation of both cigarette smoking and tuberculosis occurs during the early years of life; the morbid consequences of both usually follow decades later. Both conditions cluster in families.[16] Both occur more frequently in urban areas. Both are often associated with crowding, stress, and migration. And the two conditions usually are transmitted through intimate person-to-person contact. Both show a graded dose response relationship with respect to morbidity and mortality. Both interact strongly with other causes of chronic pulmonary disease. Both depend heavily upon social factors; both are epidemic in nature. With cigarette smoking, the mode of spread is not the airborne transmission of bacteria, but rather the transmission of a learned behavior reinforced by the pharmacological effects of nicotine.

To find risk groups for cigarette smoking, one can look among the preadolescent population for those who identify with toughness, for those who are impetuous, for those who are sexually precocious, and for those who are not doing well in school.[17] Also at high risk to being smokers are those whose friends, older siblings, and/or parents are cigarette smokers.[18]

One interesting difference from tuberculosis is that the extinction of the condition, cessation of smoking, is also transmissible from person to person. Thus, the counterepidemic can compete successfully and perhaps even overwhelm the primary epidemic, smoking.

2. Regularly Reported

After the U.S. Surgeon General's 1963 report on cigarette smoking, the Current Population Survey began to interview about cigarette smoking on a national basis, undertaking surveys for 1964, 1966, and yearly thereafter.[19] The principal forms of regional, state, and local data that are available on a population basis derive from taxes on cigarettes and represent rough and incomplete information. But the collection of preventive and therapeutic data concerning cigarettte smoking on a population basis is nonexistent. No intelligence about smoking exists comparable to that from the tuberculosis case register which describes those who have the problem, those who are receiving treatment or preventive services, and what success has been obtained. The mandatory reporting of cigarette smoking would be socially unacceptable, yet many smokers and many of their physicians might choose to use a well-organized means of following over time the individuals' smoking habits. An ongoing assessment of preventive efforts is only possible by following the population over time to see if those receiving the services smoke less often than those who don't receive them. Today it is as important to know the percentage of sixth, ninth, and twelfth graders who smoke cigarettes as it is to know their tuberculosis skin-test status.

3. Diagnostic Standards

The basic classification of cigarette smokers—by numbers of cigarettes smoked per day—has served well the studies correlating smoking with morbidity and mortality, and even in this regard pleas have been issued for more refined assessment of total tar and nicotine dosage.[20] But dosage factors do not provide the clinician direct clues as to how the smoking behavior should be managed clinically. . . . Is this a person who wants to give up cigarette smoking? What therapeutic measures will be most likely to work? What ecological factors must be considered here? Is this patient a high priority person epidemiologically, i.e., in terms of others' smoking?

Not only do we need an assessment of knowledge, attitudes, and motivation of the individual smoker, but we likewise need a systematic view of the smoker's social environment. Do the spouse, friends, or work associates smoke? Does the smoker have distinct periods of pressure or anxiety tied to smoking? What places serve as cues to smoking?

Despite the completion of many cohort studies of the morbidity and mortality of cigarette smoking, there is urgent need for a cohort study based upon presmoking (childhood and family) behavior, with the outcome variable being the cigarette smoking itself. From such studies we will learn more about who is at high risk for smoking and what are the circumstances which initiate the habit.

4. Prevention Rigorously Evaluated

The reported results of health education campaigns against smoking are disappointing on two counts: (a) their methods and follow-up often have been wanting (many had no control groups and even more did not report long-term results); and (b) the results are universally disappointing, with little or no decrease in smoking.[21] At least one study is trying to assess prevention on a community level and to evaluate carefully the results—the Stanford Heart Disease Prevention Program.[22]

5. Treatment Rigorously Evaluated

Several reviews have summarized the treatment of behavioral problems in preventive medicine, cigarette smoking in particular.[23] Without rigorous studies which spell out the long-term benefits and the costs of alternative forms of treatment, we are handicapped in deciding which are the best programs to choose for inducing cessation and which elements of these programs are vital. It is clear however that two ingredients, knowledge of the risk of smoking and will power, are insufficient to change the behavior of the overwhelming majority of smokers. Yet this is the strategy pursued by many responsible persons, both lay and professional. Treatment will be far more successful when it is broadly recognized that the cessation of smoking is for most smokers a complex behavioral process requiring time, repeated effort, and the proper social milieu.[24]

In comparison to the large scale, multicenter studies of the treatment of tuberculosis, few national resources have been committed to the evaluation of methods of treatment of cigarette smoking. Various aspects of treatment must be specified, such as initial source of patient, eligibility for treatment, diagnosis of smoking pattern, specification of treatment and adjunctive measures, criteria for success (preferably complete cessation of cigarette smoking), and follow-up intervals.[25]

6. Social And Psychological Factors

Most studies which have examined the personal characteristics of cigarette smokers compared to nonsmokers have shown no clearcut evidence identifying either a distinct smoker's personality or characteristics that are pathological.[26] Nevertheless, behavioral differences exist between cigarette smokers and nonsmokers which do set them apart.[27] The image of smoking to adolescents, whether smoker cr nonsmoker, tends to be the same: the smoker is seen to be impulsive, tough, sexually precocious, and not very successful in school. The impulsiveness seems to extend into adult life in several ways. High and excessive alcohol consumption is strongly correlated with cigarette smoking.[28] Cigarette smokers are involved in more than their share of accidents.[29] And male cigarette smokers have been found to underutilize physician and dental services compared to male never-smokers.[30]

One of the striking, and little understood features of cigarette smoking is the degree of social segregation which surrounds it.[31] The friends of smokers overwhelmingly tend to smoke, and the friends of nonsmokers don't smoke. The cigarette undoubtedly serves as the badge of membership for some adolescent groups and as a ban to others. Adults also show social segregation according to smoking status, though the partitioning is not as dramatic as that found in adolescence.[32] The significance of the induction into cigarette smoking by one's peers may last longer than is generally recognized. Tobacco is often called the smoker's friend and, in times of distress or loneliness, this friend often provides a source of comfort and pleasure.

Once the smoking has become habitual, any of a number of stimuli may lead the person to light up. There are the so-called negative-affect smokers who smoke in response to feelings of anger, depression, and frustration; the positive-affect smokers who smoke when they're feeling good; the habitual smoker who may not even be aware he or she is lighting up—no decision is made to smoke; and the social smoker, the one who lights up when offered a cigarette and in the company of other smokers.[33]

Giving up cigarettes has been traced to several kinds of circumstances and motivations. One of the foremost is the development of symptoms or the receipt of advice from a doctor not to smoke. Another common reason has to do with the need to master one's own behavior, to be more powerful than the cigarette. Other reasons are given less often: the expense, the unappealing ashes and smell, bad breath and decreased allure, and escape from the badgering of friends and relatives.

In the literature on the natural history of smoking, two types of studies are scarce—cohort studies among youngsters which seek to identify events that lead to the initiation and cessation of smoking.[34] Who are the highly contagious smokers, who infect (initiate) many of the susceptibles about them with the habit? What are the prior characteristics of those who take up the habit and those who turn it down? What are the characteristics of the situations where successful transmission occurs and those where it fails? What is the incubation period, that is the time from initial exposure (or exposures) until the time the youngster is habituated? How do adolescent subgroups, cliques, and social standing affect the initiation of smoking?

And concerning cessation: How do the known factors associated with cessation impinge on the regular smoker before he or she decides to forego the habit? What is the distribution of attempts to give up the habit before success is finally met? What are the emotional and other costs of attempting to give up the habit? Can we identify types of regular smokers who are particularly suited to particular approaches to cessation?

The research that is required must be oriented toward the behavioral dynamics of the starting and stopping of cigarette smoking. Characteristics and attitudes of persons are interesting, but they may tell us more about how persons respond to a questionnaire than about their behavior and feelings when actually confronting their cigarette smoking.

7. Societal Responsibility

Over the last decade the U.S. federal government has taken certain measures against cigarette smoking on a societal level.[35] Information which describes the hazards of cigarette smoking has been broadly distributed. Health educators have sought to use attitude change in addition to information about the hazards of cigarettes to diminish the frequency of smoking in the population. But overall, the consumption of cigarettes has changed relatively little, decreasing slightly in men and increasing among women.[36] Unlike the tuberculosis bacillus, cigarettes have articulate and skillful advocates, many of whom have an economic incentive to propagate smoking.[37]

At the institutional level, we find no agency which has assumed responsibility for controlling cigarette smoking. When a dangerous epidemic rages, which here is the case, who should bear the onus for containing the epidemic, for maximizing the number of smokers who convert to nonsmokers? Is the responsible agency to be the health department? At present, few local health departments have seriously engaged in therapeutic antismoking activites. Will health maintenance organizations be the responsible agency? Few of the population receive care from health maintenance organizations, and very few health maintenance organizations try to modify cigarette smoking systematically.[38]

Two kinds of agencies have been most committed to smoking cessation, the voluntary health organizations (Action for Smoking and Health, Group Against Smoking Pollution, the American Heart Association, the American Lung Association, and the American Cancer Society) and certain federal health agencies (the U.S. Public Health Service and the National Clearinghouse on Smoking and Health).

At the societal level two social forces can be identified which are likely to affect cigarette consumption—the generation gap and the unceasing crescendo of medical care costs.

To the extent that the onset of smoking reflects adolescent rebellion, and to the extent that youth or some segment of youth feels alienated from the older generation, so a substantial fraction of youngsters will be inducted into the habit of smoking. Perhaps the more cigarettes are identified by adult society as dangerous and harmful, the more they will be taken up by at least the disenchanted segment of youth. For the alienated, it would seem that the message about cigarette smoking might be delivered most effectively by a fellow alien. Though some attempts to decrease cigarette consumption through a peer approach have been tried, we find no rigorous studies which evaluate the results.

With U.S. health care costs rising to $104,239,000,000 in 1973 and with increasing public financing of medical care, the extra medical costs generated by cigarette smoking will come under increasingly heavy attack.[39] Several studies have shown that cigarette smokers use disproportionately high quantities of the most expensive services—those associated with hospitalization.[40] As has already been proposed in some quarters, there will be pressure to tax cigarettes for the excess medical costs which they generate.[41] This might lead to differential premiums for smokers and nonsmokers. In any case, the expenditures of the medical care sector will add further fuel to the anticigarette fire.

8. Defined Targets For The System

Once a method of treating cigarette smoking is shown to be measurably effective, the consequences of applying the treatment to those who might benefit can be calculated. Following this, population-wide targets for providing preventive care can be developed both in terms of the numbers to receive and to respond to treatment and in terms of the ultimate effect upon the future incidence and prevalence of the condition and its morbid consequences.

It is striking that we have no national targets in relation to cigarette smoking. Today 40 percent of the population is smoking. In 1985, should that percentage be 30, 20, or 10? If 20 percent of women today take up the habit by age 20, should that percentage ten years from now be halved, quartered? We in the United States have no declaration of intent about cigarette smoking. Without defining goals which we can fail to achieve, we also eliminate our chance to win real success. Furthermore, once we define population-wide targets, alternative means of accomplishing them can be explored. For example, how should resources be allocated among a mass-media approach that converts a small percentage of middle-aged smokers to nonsmokers per year, a group therapy approach which converts half of the interested smokers (but which is very expensive), and a public school approach which is found to have lasting, long-range effects on a tiny percentage of adolescents?

By defining to the public population-level goals for smoking and by offering to the public feedback on how they are progressing toward these goals, we can offer substantial support to the counterepidemic, to those who feel they have a stake in the social and economic costs of smoking. This nation seems to thrive on statistics, on news bad and good, and on social change; why not use these proclivities to further the nation's health?

To evaluate progress toward population-based goals, the cigarette registry and periodic surveys of smoking behavior are necessary. Cigarette smoking cannot become a condition which the physician, by law, will be required to report. Nevertheless, there is no way to learn how cigarette control is progressing other than to define a sample of the population, and to assess and reassess its smoking over time.

Who should set targets and priorities for preventive care? This nation has yet to formulate clear-cut policy even with respect to the provision of medical care, so, undoubtedly, it will take longer to arrive at policy for preventive services; these are much less in demand. The Department of Health, Education, and Welfare has been planning at least one major step forward. In June 1975, a major conference on prevention will be held at the Fogarty International Center which will attempt to identify what national policy should be with respect to prevention in the United States for the years 1976–80.[42] To the extent that operationally defined targets are generated by this conference and machinery set up for monitoring progress toward those targets, the nation will not need a special organization to tend prevention.

Who will play the role for smoking that the American Thoracic Society has played for tuberculosis—setting standards for prevention, diagnosis, treatment, and screening; demonstrating methods of program evaluation; and educating physicians, nurses, and technicians? There are two candidate organizations on the horizon, the American Public Health Association and the American College of Preventive Medicine. The work to be done is formidable and will take a high level of organizational commitment to preventive health care.

9. Ethical And Legal Issues

The ethical issues in pursuing cigarette smoking on a population basis are numerous, complex, and difficult. But they must not be ignored, nor the subject ignored because of them. How can we see to it that the smokers who are potential clients of our programs have a clear option to participate or to refuse? Should economic or social incentives be used to encourage cessation of cigarette smoking, and, if so, what are their limits? What are the hazards and hidden costs of trying to minimize a population's cigarette smoking? Should taxes be added to the price of cigarettes to place them out of reach of most consumers or to attempt to recoup some of the money lost to excess health care costs?

No attempt will be made to answer these questions here, but it is important they be addressed by thoughtful, responsible persons who represent diverse roles and points of view.

10. Relation To Conventional Medical Care

In seeking to curb cigarette smoking by working through primary medical care, we find a preliminary complication. Physicians are accustomed to the patient bringing them symptoms or problems which the patient finds bothersome. Physicians are not accustomed to assuming the initiative in defining the patient's problems. But precisely this is necessary in the pursuit of cigarette smoking and in many other aspects of preventive medicine. In fact, the general public expects their physicians to initiate cigarette cessation activities, but judging from patients' reports, few physicians pursue the subject systematically and vigorously.[43] The situation is reminiscent of the sporadic use of tuberculin testing in office and hospital practice in years gone by, when tuberculosis was common. Furthermore, most physicians have not been trained in behavioral methods and some find dealing with behavioral problems too boring, cumbersome, or emotionally threatening. The question arises: Should the physician be assigned the principal role in programs aimed at preventive behavior? On the one hand, patients expect their physician to be their counselor with respect to matters of health. On the other hand, many physicians have neither the time, the temperament, nor the expertise to add the demands of anticigarette counseling to their workload. At this point in time, the answer is not clear-cut. Psychologists often have better background and training for dealing with chronic behavioral problems, but some primary care physicians can be very effective counselors. Certainly, within any organized system of health care, at the clinical level, there needs to be the knowledge, the skill, and the organization to pursue preventive behavioral problems systematically. In today's medicine, as specialized as it is, this undoubtedly means having as part of the staff preventive technicians or medical specialists who can deliver preventive care adequately.

The hospital also makes an excellent site for initiating programs of cigarette-smoking cessation.[44] Smokers, when faced with a tangible worsening of their physical health, are more likely to give up the habit. In fact, there is no group that matches the short-term rate of cessation of midde-aged men recovering from myocardial infarction. One study compared the systematic counseling by a nurse practitioner of patients recovering from myocardial infarction to whatever counseling is routine for that condition. At eight months after hospital discharge, the respective rates of successful cessation were 63 percent and 45 percent for the counseled and routine groups.[45] Since ill health is highly motivating towards cessation and since ill health sharply increases the likelihood of hospitalization, counseling in hospitals should prove highly productive in terms of short-term patient cooperation. How much long-term abstinence from cigarettes is achieved and how much this group benefits from cessation as compared to smokers who do not have this much morbidity will have to await further study.

CONCLUSIONS

Like other high risk behaviors, cigarette smoking is now epidemic with respect to its effects upon health. As an epidemic condition, with identifiable risk factors, with a definable natural history, with effective treatment, and with preventive potential, the consequences of cigarette smoking warrant an approach similar to the way any other serious epidemic would be handled. This implies working at the population level in addition to an individual, case-by-case approach.

First, the agencies or health professionals who have responsibility for offering preventive care should be identified, given the resources to begin their work, and held accountable for the results. Whether they be health departments, hospitals, HMOs, or whatever, both the responsible agency and the public should recognize that an epidemic exists and recognize their separate responsibilities for its management.

Second, when institutional responsibilities have been defined, some realistic, achievable, population-based targets with respect to the incidence and prevalence of the behavior will facilitate planning for the future, allocating resources, and evaluating progress. To help achieve these targets, experts in the field should define terminology; recommend diagnostic, therapeutic, and preventive methods; and order the priority of work to be done. By spelling out the details of what is involved in the control of cigarette smoking, health care providers will share a clear idea of what is to be done and how others approach the problem.

Third, follow-up of entire segments of the population is a key factor in the control of unhealthful behaviors, just as follow-up has been central in the control of tuberculosis. Therefore, population-based registers of cigarette smokers, of groups at high risk of starting smoking, and of former smokers who may start to smoke again are essential. As with tuberculosis, it will likely be the case that persons who have successfully been treated and then followed without relapse for a certain number of years will have such a low risk of future relapse that they could be dropped from follow-up. But for those who continue to smoke, just as for persons with active tuberculosis, ongoing follow-up would offer the latest methods and benefits of treatment.

Fourth, the determinative factors in any epidemic of unhealthful behavior such as cigarette smoking are not the repeated behaviors themselves. Rather, the causal factors must be viewed as the behavioral context—the stimuli, associations, reinforcements—which transform the everyday situations faced by all persons into specific cues for the behavior. For cigarette smoking, the cup of coffee after breakfast, tension at work, or the visit of a friend may cue the smoker either to light a cigarette or to undertake an alternative behavior. Learning to do the latter consistently and reliably is what cessation of smoking is about. Thus, cessation of cigarette smoking is primarily a newly learned set of responses and not an exercise of will, of intelligence, or of magic.

Fifth, and finally, to the extent that preventive medicine seeks to meddle with the intimate, personal behaviors of the population on a mass basis, we need to have before us the thoughtful deliberation of the ethical and legal considerations which should frame our work. We wish to contribute to the health of the population, not to aggravate feelings of guilt or failure nor to punish those who freely choose the unhealthful behavior after considering the alternatives. But to argue that no one has the right to meddle in personal matters such as smoking is to ignore the forces which market, advertise, promote, and distribute cigarettes. The advertiser's appeal to power, prowess, privacy, beauty, humor are all attempts to insert into our everyday behavior the name of, and the need for, a particular kind of cigarette. This careful and skillful meddling with our personal behavior warrants some humane, countervailing force.

The final argument for action comes from those who have successfully given up their unhealthful behavior—despite the tension and struggle necessary to overcome the habit, despite missing the pleasure and satisfaction of the old behavior, the great majority of former smokers delight in their success at having foresaken smoking. In three words: It feels good!

NOTES

1. O. Pomerleau, F. Bass, and V. Crown, "The Role of Behavior Modification in Preventive Medicine," *New England Journal of Medicine* (forthcoming).

2. B. MacMahon, T. F. Pugh, and J. Ipsen, *Epidemiologic Methods* (Boston: Little, Brown, & Co., 1960).

3. A. S. Pope and J. E. Gordon, "The Impact of Tuberculosis on Human Populations," *American Journal of Medical Science,* vol. 230, 1955, pp. 317–53.

4. M. L. Atkinson, "A New Method for the Evaluation of Tuberculosis Control Programs," *Health Services Reports,* vol. 88, 1973, pp. 489–92.

5. American Lung Association, *Diagnostic Standards and Classification of Tuberculosis* (New York: American Lung Association, 1974).

6. J. B. Shaw and N. Wynn Williams, "Infectivity of Pulmonary Tuberculosis in Relation to Sputum Status," *American Review of Respiratory Diseases,* vol. 69, 1954, pp. 724–27.

7. E. C. Chamberlayne, ed., *Status of Immunization in Tuberculosis in 1971*, DHEW Publ., 72–68, Bethesda, 1972.

8. National Tuberculosis Association, "Chemoprophylaxis for the Prevention of Tuberculosis: A Statement by an Ad Hoc Committee," *American Review of Respiratory Diseases*, vol. 96, 1967, pp. 558–60.

9. National Tuberculosis Association, "Standards for Tuberculosis Treatment in the 1970's: A Statement by an Ad Hoc Committee," *American Review of Respiratory Diseases*, vol. 96, 1967, pp. 558–60.

10. T. Moulding, "New Responsibilities for Health Departments and Public Health Nurses in Tuberculosis: Keeping the Outpatient on Therapy," *American Journal of Public Health*, vol. 56, 1966, pp. 416-25.

11. F. Bass, *Guidelines for the Outpatient Care of Tuberculosis in New Jersey* (Trenton, N.J.: State of New Jersey Department of Health, 1964).

12. Atkinson, "A New Method for the Evaluation of Tuberculosis Control Programs."

13. National Tuberculosis Association, "Bacteriologic Standards for the Discharge of Patients: A Statement by the Committee on Bacteriologic Standards for the Discharge of Patients, American Thoracic Society," *American Review of Respiratory Diseases*, vol 102, December 1970.

14. American Lung Association of Southeastern Michigan, "Evaluation of the Tuberculosis Control Program for Detroit and Wayne County" October 16, 1974 (Detroit: Lung Association, 1974).

15. National Tuberculosis Association, "Infectiousness of Tuberculosis: A Report of the NTA Ad Hoc Committee on Treatment of Tb patients in General Hospitals," *American Review of Respiratory Diseases*, vol. 96, October 1967.

16. J. M. Bynner, *The Young Smoker: A Study of Smoking among Schoolboys Carried Out for the Ministry of Health*, Government Social Survey SS 383 (London: Her Majesty's Stationery Office, 1969).

17. Ibid., S. V. Zagona, ed., *Studies and Issues in Smoking Behavior* (Tucson: University of Arizona Press, 1967).

18. Ibid.

19. U.S., Department of Health, Education, and Welfare, *Current Estimates from the Health Interview Survey: United States, 1971*, Vital & Health Statistics, ser. 10, no. 79 (1973).

20. S. M. Waingrow, D. Horn, and F. F. Ikar, "Dosage Patterns of Cigarette Smoking in American Adults," *American Journal of Public Health*, vol. 58, 1968, pp. 54–70.

21. P. W. Bradshaw, "The Problem of Cigarette Smoking and Its Control," *International Journal of the Addictions*, vol. 8, 1973, pp. 353–71; W. W. Holland, and A. Elliott, "Cigarette Smoking, Respiratory Symptoms, and Anti-Smoking Propaganda," *Lancet*, vol. 1, 1968, pp. 41–43.

22. J. W. Farquhar, "Interdisciplinary Approaches to Heart Disease Prevention (Results of a Community-based Risk Reduction Campaign Using Mass Media)," paper presented to the AAAS meeting, New York, January 30, 1975 (processed).

23. J. L. Schwartz, "A Critical Review and Evaluation of Smoking Control Methods," *Public Health Reports*, vol. 84, 1969, pp. 483–506; A. McAlister, "Helping People Quit Smoking: Current Progress," in A. Enelow et al., eds., *Applying Behavioral Science to Cardiovascular Disease* (New York: American Heart Association, 1975).

24. D. A. Bernstein, "The Modification of Smoking Behavior: A Search for Effective Variables," *Behavior Research and Therapy*, vol. 8, 1970, pp. 133–46; M. J. Mahoney, "Research Issues in Self-Management," *Behavior Therapy*, vol. 3, 1972, pp. 45–63.

25. Bradshaw, "Problem of Cigarette Smoking and Its Control."

26. E. D. Borgatta and R. R. Evans, eds., *Smoking, Health, and Behavior* (Chicago: Aldine Publishing Co., 1968).

27. Zagona, ed., *Studies and Issues in Smoking Behavior*.

28. M. W. Higgins and M. Kjelsberg, "Characteristics of Smokers and Nonsmokers in Tecumseh, Michigan, II: The Distribution of Selected Physical Measurements and Physiologic Variables and the Prevalence of Certain Diseases in Smokers and Nonsmokers," *American Journal of Epidemiology,* vol. 86, 1967, pp. 60–77.

29. J. D. Matarazzo and G. Saslow, "Psychological and Related Characteristics of Smokers and Nonsmokers," *Psychological Bulletin,* vol. 57, 1960, pp. 493–513.

30. F. Bass, "Medical Care Use Attributable to Cigarette Smoking" (D.Sc. thesis, Johns Hopkins University School of Hygiene and Public Health, 1973).

31. A. C. McKennell and R. K. Thomas, *Adults' and Adolescents' Smoking Habits and Attitudes: A Report on a Survey Carried Out for the Ministry of Health,* Government Social Survey 353/B. (London: Her Majesty's Stationery Office, 1969).

32. Ibid.

33. S. Tomkins, "A Modified Model of Smoking Behavior," in Borgatta and Evans, eds., *Smoking, Health, and Behavior.*

34. Zagona, ed., *Studies and Issues in Smoking Behavior.*

35. U.S., Department of Health, Education, and Welfare, *The Consequences of Smoking,* DHEW Publ., 74–8704, Bethesda, January 1974.

36. Gallup Organization, Inc., *Survey of Cigarette Smoking, 1974* (Princeton: Gallup Organization, Inc., 1974).

37. M. Terris, "Breaking the Barriers to Prevention: Legislative Approaches," *Bulletin of the New York Academy of Medicine,* vol. 51, 1975, pp. 242–57.

38. P. B. Peacock, A. C. Gelman, and T. A. Lutins, *Preventive Health Care Strategies for Health Maintenance Organizations* (New York: American Health Foundation, 1974).

39. U.S., Department of Health, Education, and Welfare, Social Security Administration, *SRS Research & Statistics,* note no. 32: *National Health Expenditures, Fiscal Year 1974,* November 29, 1974.

40. Bass, "Medical Care Use Attributable to Cigarette Smoking."

41. R. M. Veatch and P. Steinfels, "Who Should Pay for Smokers' Medical Care?" *Hastings Center Report,* November 1974, pp. 8–10.

42. American College of Preventive Medicine, "National Conference on Preventive Medicine," *Newsletter of the American College of Preventive Medicine,* vol. 15, no. 4, 1974, p. 1.

43. E. Green and E. Horn, *Physicians' Attitude toward Their Involvement in Smoking Problems of Their Patients* (Arlington, Va.: U.S. National Clearinghouse for Smoking and Health, 1968).

44. K. Ball, "Hospital Beds and Cigarette Smoking," *Lancet,* vol. 2, 1970, p. 48; A. Burt, D. Illingworth, T. D. R. Shaw, et al., "Stopping Smoking after Myocardial Infarction," *Lancet,* vol. 1, 1974, pp. 304–07.

45. Burt, et al., "Stopping Smoking after Myocardial Infarction."

Appendix L
Methods Available to Evaluate the Health Education Components of Preventive Health Programs

by
Lawrence W. Green, Dr.P.H.*

DEFINITION AND INCLUSIONS

The health education components of preventive health programs may be considered to include:

1. *communications* directed at the public and at patients and families to influence knowledge, attitudes, beliefs, and norms supporting health practices;

2. *community organization* activities designed to influence the voluntary adjustment of resources to make health services more accessible and acceptable to the populations in need of these services; and

3. *staff development* activities such as consultation, supervision, inservice training, and continuing education designed to influence the attitudes and behavior of providers toward patients and clients so as to reinforce appropriate health behavior in the public.[1] The common feature of these three modalities of health education, and therefore, the defining characteristics of health education strategies, is that they are designed to bring about *voluntary* changes in health-related behavior. This distinguishes educational strategies from legal, administrative, environmental control, political, medical, and other strategies, although health education may be used in support of these alternative strategies.

*Associate Professor of Public Health Administration and Head, Division of Health Education, Johns Hopkins University School of Hygiene and Public Health, Baltimore, Maryland.

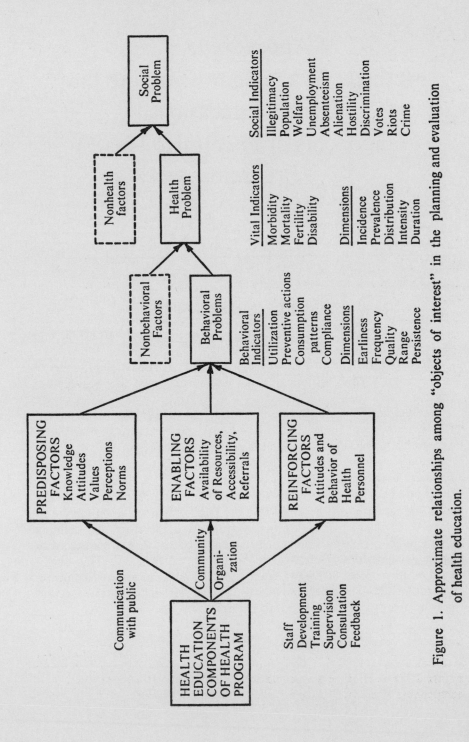

Figure 1. Approximate relationships among "objects of interest" in the planning and evaluation of health education.

1234567

EDUCATIONAL INPUT (Cost)	BEHAVIORAL OUTCOME	MEDICAL OR ADMINISTRATIVE BENEFIT
Showing concern and interest for needs of the patient or population	Patient satisfaction	Public support for the program or agency Payment of bills by patients Reduced malpractice suits Kept appointments (reduced broken appointments) Competitive with quacks and other alternatives
Communication of information	Patient knowledge, attitudes, beliefs	Compliance, better diagnosis
Entertainment or other appeal to motives and values of the patient	Patient interest, reduced boredom	Reduced delay, kept appointments
Communication with relatives	Social support for patient	Compliance, public support
Outreach	Public awareness, interest, attitudes, preventive health behavior	Patient recruitment, primary prevention, appropriate utilization
In-Service training	Staff awareness, interest, attitudes, showing concern	Patient satisfaction, patient knowledge (see above)
Community organization	Coordination of resources, referrals; social support for patients	Appropriate utilization, patient recruitment, reduced duplication, public support
Mass communication	Public awareness, interest, some social support, some knowledge	Public support, patient recruitment, reduced delay
Follow-up contact with former patients	Patient reinforcement, sustained interest and commitment	return appointments, continued adoption persistence, compliance)

Figure 2. Theoretical relationships between some specific educational components of a health program and the expected benefits.

OUTCOMES MEASURED IN THE EVALUATION OF HEALTH EDUCATION

The immediate outcomes of the three health education modalities are identified in Figure 1 as:

1. *predisposing* factors,
2. *enabling* factors, and
3. *reinforcing* factors.

These factors are viewed as antecedent to behavioral changes which are sought in preventive health programs. Indicators and dimensions of behavioral measurement for the evaluation of health education outcomes are listed below "Behavioral Problems" in Figure 1. Measures of the more immediate (antecedent) variables to the left provide "process" evaluation in health education.[2]

INPUT MEASUREMENT IN EVALUATION OF HEALTH EDUCATION

Because behavioral changes are dependent on a variety of antecedent variables (predisposing, enabling, and reinforcing factors), each of which must be influenced by a distinct educational input, the evaluation of health education *programs* or strategies must be distinguished from evaluation of specific health education techniques or tactics. The latter may be related on a theoretical level with the specific outcomes each is expected to influence, as in Figure 2, but the outcomes are maximized in practice by the *combination* of various inputs.[3] These and related considerations in the design of health education programs have implications for the appropriate adaptation and analysis of experimental and quasi-experimental designs to evaluate health education.[4] The measurement of inputs must similarly take into account factors specific to the educational process and educational technology, such as the usual relationship between unit costs and effectiveness,[5] economies of scale in informational technologies,[6] the logarithmic diffusion curve in the penetration of community programs,[7] the quality of educational media,[8] personnel used,[9] and the setting and circumstances of the educational encounter or exposure.[10]

The methods and instruments to measure these input variables have been variously developed but are far from standardized except where simple counts are possible, as in the number of pamphlets distributed, number of home visits made, hours of mass media time used, etc.[11]

MEASURING PREBEHAVIORAL OUTCOMES OF HEALTH EDUCATION

There are widely standardized measurement instruments available for some health-related knowledge inventories and attitude scales. Unfortunately, the better standardized tools tend to measure the least important health beliefs and attitudes. The most documented set of health beliefs known to be related to a variety of health behaviors, for example, are almost totally without standardization and tests of reliability or of validity.[12] Knowledge inventories and attitude scales are relatively well standardized, on the other hand, in trivial areas by health behavior criteria.[13] Personality measures are the most extensively and thoroughly tested and standardized scales,[14] but fail repeatedly to explain more than a tenth of the variance in most health behaviors, with the notable exception of the internal-external "Locus of Control" scale[15] and possibly the "Value Orientation" scale.[16] Measures of predisposing demographic variables are better standardized than psychological variables, with most of the standardization following U.S. Census Bureau procedures, but some being adapted to reflect social psychological predispositions or to maximize the variance accounted for in health behavior.[17] Measures of relative *exposure* and *reactions* to various mass media, such as the Nielsen ratings, are well developed.[18]

Community organization outcomes are the most difficult to evaluate in most health education programs because of the difficulty of controlling extraneous factors influencing the outcomes. Case studies have been the major source of evaluative information,[19] particularly in the analysis of interorganizational relationships.[20] Considerable efforts in recent years have yielded new methods and procedures for measuring process and outcomes of consumer participation in health planning.[21] Another influence of community organization on enabling factors that has received increased methodological development is health referral patterns.[22]

Staff development outcomes are now receiving increased attention with the growing interest in continuing education and new manpower configurations in health services. Evaluation of training programs and of supervision has traditionally been limited to "reactionnaires" asking trainees or supervisors how they liked various aspects of their supervisor or the training program.[23] The gradual adoption of more formal use of task analysis and instructional objectives by trainers has given impetus and greater feasibility to the evaluation of behavioral outcomes in training and supervision.[24] These developments have also improved the prospects for evaluation of consultation[25] and of institutional and continuing education.[26]

From the standpoint of health education in preventive health programs, the *process* to which these staff development activities are addressed is improved attitudes and behavior of staff toward patients. Instruments focused specifically on these process variables are emerging in a variety of contexts.[27]

MEASURING BEHAVIORAL OUTCOMES OF HEALTH EDUCATION

Standardized measures of behavioral outcomes are better developed than measures of the antecedent and process variables discussed above, but agreement on methods and procedures for collecting, analyzing, and interpreting behavioral measures is far from unanimous. The most extensive methodological work has been with indices of health service utilization.[28] Recent reviews of the literature, however, reveal wide discrepancies on criteria of "adequate" or "appropriate" utilization in terms of delay[29] and the frequency or duration of return appointments.[30]

Greater discrepancies are found in the measurement of preventive health practices,[31] in compliance with medical regimens,[32] and in risk-reduction behavior (screening tests, smoking, weight control, diet, etc.).[33] The overlap among these behavioral categories is part of the problem, but the lack of agreement on measures of behavior within categories is not eliminated by reclassification.

IMPLICATIONS FOR FUTURE EVALUATION OF HEALTH EDUCATION

The major obstacle to advancing the scientific base of health education practice in preventive health programs is clearly the paucity of standardized measures of both input and outcome variables. This precludes the comparison of findings between studies and limits the generalizability of results. The scientific and professional literature related to health education is mushrooming in both the behavioral science and the health science journals, but it lacks the cumulative quality essential to the codification of knowledge and the development of theory and policy.

These conclusions lead to a major recommendation for governmental action to encourage methodological research on the measurement of health education variables and the standardization of instruments to improve the comparability of findings from various studies. A second recommendation should be to increase support for replicative studies. Most grants and contracts have been for isolated, ad hoc studies, rather than for evaluative research *programs* in which the same educational strategies are retested in different settings or with carefully controlled variations.

Notes
1. L. W. Green, "Toward Cost-Benefit Evaluations of Health Education: Some Concepts, Methods, and Examples," *Health Education Monographs*, vol. 2, supp. 1, May 1974, pp. 34-60.
2. Ibid.
3. Ibid.
4. L. W. Green and I. Figa-Talamanca, "Suggested Designs for Evaluation of Health Education Programs," *Health Education Monographs*, vol. 2, Spring 1974, pp. 54-71; L. W. Green, D. M. Levine, and S. Deeds, "Clinical Trials of Health Education for Hypertensive Outpatients: Design and Baseline Data," paper presented to the Eastern Section of the American Federation for Clinical Research, January 1975.

5. L. W. Green, "Cost Containment and the Economics of Health Education in Medical Care," *Hospitals, the Journal of the American Hospital Association*, vol. 49, 1975.

6. A. G. Oetlinger and N. Zapol, "Will Information Technologies Help Learning?" *Teachers College Record*, vol. 74, September 1972, pp. 5–54.

7. Green, "Toward Cost-Benefit Evaluations of Health Education"; L. W. Green, "Diffusion and Adoption of Innovations Related to Cardiovascular Risk Behavior in the Public," in A. Enelow, J. Henderson, and E. Berkanovic, eds., *Applying Behavioral Sciences to Cardiovascular Risk* (New York: American Heart Association, 1975).

8. P. L. Campeau, "Selective Review of the Results of Research on the Use of Audiovisual Media to Teach Adults," *AV Communications Review*, vol. 22, Spring 1974, pp. 5–40; S. G. Deeds, "Promises! Promises! Educational Technology for Health Education Audiences," paper presented to the annual meeting of the American Public Health Association, San Francisco, 1973.

9. Green, "Diffusion and Adoption of Innovations Related to Cardiovascular Risk Behavior in the Public"; S. R. Fletcher, "A Study of the Effectiveness of a Follow-up Clerk in an Emergency Room" (M.Sc. thesis, Johns Hopkins University School of Hygiene and Public Health, 1973); J. B. Atwater, "Adapting the Venereal Disease Clinic to Today's Problems," *American Journal of Public Health*, vol. 64, May 1974, pp. 433–37; W. R. Cuskey and T. Prekumer, "A Differential Role Model for the Treatment of Drug Addicts," *Health Services Reports*, vol. 88, 1973, pp. 663-68; D. M. Tagliacozzo et al., "Nurse Intervention and Patient Behavior: An Experimental Study," *American Journal of Public Health*, vol. 64, June 1974, pp. 596–603; S. P. Rosenzweig and R. Folman, "Patient and Therapist Variables Affecting Premature Termination in Group Psychotherapy," *Psychotherapy: Theory, Research and Practice*, vol. 11, Spring 1974, pp. 76–79; B. Freemon et al., "Gaps in Doctor-Patient Communications: Doctor-Patient Interaction Analysis," *Pediatric Research*, vol. 5, 1971, pp. 298–311.

10. L. W. Green, "Should Health Education Abandon Attitude Change Strategies: Perspectives from Recent Research," *Health Education Monographs*, vol. 1, no. 30, 1970, pp. 25–48.

11. E. L. Baker and M. C. Alkin, "ERIC/AVCR Annual Review Paper: Formative Evaluation of Instructional Development," *AV Communication Review*, vol. 21, Winter 1973, pp. 389–418.

12. M. H. Baker, ed., "Personal Health Practices and the Health Belief Model," *Health Education Monographs*, vol. 2, Winter 1974, pp. 324–473.

13. R. B. Cattell, "How Good is the Modern Questionnaire? General Principles of Evaluation," *Journal of Personality Assessment*, vol. 38, April 1974, pp. 115–29.

14. G. M. Maranell, ed., *Scaling: A Sourcebook for Behavioral Scientists* (Chicago: Aldine Publishing Co., 1974).

15. J. Schopler et al., "The North Carolina Internal-External Scale: Validation of the Short Form," *Research Previews*, vol. 20, November 1973, pp. 3–12.

16. L. Mezei, "Factorial Validity of the Kluckhohn and Strodtbeck Value Orientation Scale," *Journal of Social Psychology*, vol. 92, February 1974, pp. 145–46.

17. L. W. Green, *Status Identity and Preventive Health Behavior*, Pacific Health Education Reports, no. 1 (Berkeley: University of California, 1970); L. W. Green, "Manual for Scoring Socioeconomic Status for Research on Health Behavior," *Public Health Reports*, vol. 85, September 1970, pp. 815–27; D. Coburn and Clyde R. Pope, "Socioeconomic Status and Preventive Health Behavior," *Journal of Health and Social Behavior*, vol. 15, June 1974, pp. 67–78; J. Saunders, J. M. Davis, and D. M. Monsees, "Opinion Leadership in Family Planning," *Journal of Health and Social Behavior*, vol. 15, September 1974, pp. 217–27; A. A. Fisher, "The Predictive Validity of a Measure of Opinion Leadership in Family Planning," *Health Education Monographs*, vol. 3, Summer 1975.

18. R. L. Stevenson, "Cross-Cultural Validation of a Readership Prediction Technique," *Journalism Quarterly*, vol. 50, Winter 1973, pp. 690–96; F. B. Collen and K. Soghikian, "Health Exhibits Accentuate the Positive," *Hospitals, the Journal of the American Hospital Association*, vol. 48, March 16, 1974, pp. 92–95; J. A. Czepiel, "Word-of-Mouth Processes in the Diffusion of a Major Technological Innovation," *Journal of Marketing Research*, vol. 11, May 1974, pp. 172–80; J. R. Lynn, "Perception of Public Service Advertising: Source, Message and Receiver Effects," *Journalism Quarterly*, vol. 50, Winter 1973, pp. 673–79, 689; A. W. Thornton, "Mass Communications and Dental Health Behavior," *Health Education Monographs*, vol. 2, Fall 1974, pp. 201–08;

19. J. N. Kerri, "Anthropological Studies of Voluntary Associations and Voluntary Action: A Review," *Journal of Voluntary Action Research*, vol. 3, January 1974, pp. 10–25.

20. P. E. White and G. T. Vlasak, *Interorganizational Research in Health: Bibliography (1960–70)*, DHEW Publ. (HSM) 72–3028, Washington, D.C., 1972.

21. J. M. Metsch and J. E. Veney, "Measuring the Outcome of Consumer Participation," *Journal of Health and Social Behavior*, vol. 14, December 1973, pp. 368–74; A. K. Tomeh, "Formal Voluntary Organizations: Participation, Correlates and Interrelationships," *Sociological Inquiry*, vol. 43, 1973, pp. 89–122; K. B. Partridge, "Community and Professional Participation in Decision-Making at a Health Center, *Health Services Reports*, vol. 88, June-July 1973, pp. 527–34.

22. J. G. Cauffman et al., "A Study of Health Referral Patterns," *American Journal of Public Health*, vol. 64, April 1974, pp. 331–56.

23. W. S. Blumenfeld and D. P. Crane, "Opinions of Training Effectiveness: How Good?" *Training and Development Journal*, vol. 27, December 1973, pp. 42–51; B. Gaoni, "Supervision from the Point of View of the Supervisee," *American Journal of Psychotherapy*, vol. 28, January 1974, pp. 108–14.

24. E. Viano, "The Styles of Management Inventory: A Methodological Analysis of a Training and Research Instrument," *Quality and Quantification*, vol. 7, 1973, pp. 91–106; C. J. Vander Kolk, "Comparison of Two Mental Health Counselor Training Programs," *Community Mental Health Journal*, vol. 9, Fall 1973, pp. 260–69; M. K. Goin, "Supervision Observed," *Journal of Nervous and Mental Diseases*, vol. 158, March 1974, pp. 208–13.

25. P. S. Stephenson, "Judging the Effectiveness of a Consultation Program to a Community Agency," *Community Mental Health Journal*, vol. 9, Fall 1973, pp. 253–59.

26. D. M. Levine and A. J. Bonito, "Impact of Clinical Training on Attitudes of Medical Students: Self-Perpetuating Barrier to Change in the System," *British Journal of Medical Education*, vol. 8, March 1974, pp. 13–16; C. White, "Patient Characteristics and Supportive Behavior of Nursing Personnel in Nursing Homes" (Dr. P. H. diss., Johns Hopkins University School of Hygiene and Public Health, 1973); T. S. Inui, "Effects of Post-Graduate Physician Education on the Management and Outcomes of Patients with Hypertension" (M. Sc. thesis, Johns Hopkins University School of Hygiene and Public Health, 1973); R. L. Ebel, "Evaluation and Educational Objectives," *Journal of Educational Measurement*, vol. 10, Winter 1973, pp. 273–79.

27. Freemon, "Gaps in Doctor-Patient Communications"; White, "Patient Characteristics and Supportive Behavior of Nursing Personnel in Nursing Homes"; Inui, "Effects of Post-Graduate Physician Education on the Management and Outcomes of Patients with Hypertension"; R. M. Balaban, "The Contribution of Participant Observation to the Study of Processes in Program Evaluation," *International Journal of Mental Health*, vol. 2, Summer 1973, pp. 59–70; K. W. Carlson, "Increasing Verbal Empathy as a Function of Feedback and Instruction," *Counselor Education and Supervision*, vol. 13, March 1974, p. 208; C. M. Rossiter, "The Use of Video-

tape Recordings in Teaching Interpersonal Communications," *Speech Teacher*, vol. 23, January 1974, pp. 59–60; S. H. Surlin, "Broadcasters' Misperceptions of Black Community Needs," *Journal of Black Studies*, vol. 4, December 1973, pp. 185–93; L. Pankratz and D. Pankratz, "Nursing Autonomy and Patients' Rights: Development of a Nursing Attitude Scale," *Journal of Health and Social Behavior*, vol. 15, September 1974, pp. 211–16.

28. L. A. Aday and R. Eichorn, *The Utilization of Health Services—Indices and Correlates: A Research Bibliography*, U.S., Department of Health, Education, and Welfare, National Center for Health Services Research and Development, DHEW Publ. (HSM) 73–3033, 1972.

29. A. Antonovsky and H. Hartman, "Delay in the Detection of Cancer: A Review of the Literature," *Health Education Monographs*, vol. 2, Summer 1974, pp. 98–128; L. W. Green and B. J. Roberts, "The Research Literature on Why Women Delay in Seeking Medical Care for Breast Symptoms," *Health Education Monographs*, vol. 2, Summer 1974, pp. 129–77.

30. E. Glogow, "Effects of Health Education Methods on Appointment Breaking," *Public Health Reports*, vol. 85, May 1970, pp. 441–50; M. R. Greenlick, D. K. Freeborn, T. J. Colombo, et al., "Comparing the Use of Medical Care Services by a Medically Indigent and a General Membership Population in a Comprehensive Prepaid Group Practice Program," *Medical Care*, vol. 10, May-June, 1972, pp. 187–200; A. V. Hurtado, M. R. Greenlick, and T. J. Colombo, "Determinants of Medical Care Utilization: Failure to Keep Appointments," *Medical Care*, vol. 11, May-June 1973, pp. 189–98; O. C. Stine, C. Chuaqui, C. Jiminez, et al., "Broken Appointments at a Comprehensive Clinic for Children," *Medical Care*, vol. 6, July-August, 1968, pp. 332–39; M. B. Sussman, E. K. Caplan, M. R. Haug, et al., *The Walking Patient: A Study in Outpatient Care* (Cleveland: The Press of Western Reserve University, 1967); J. F. Caldwell, S. Cobb, M. D. Dowling, et al., "The Dropout Problem in an Antihypertensive Treatment," *Journal of Chronic Diseases*, vol. 22, February 1970, pp. 579–92; F. A. Finnerty, Jr., E. C. Mattie, and F. A. Finnerty, III, "Hypertension in the Inner City, I: Analysis of Clinic Dropouts," *Circulation*, vol. 47, January 1973, pp. 73–75.

31. Green, *Status Identity and Preventive Health Behavior*; Coburn and Pope, "Socioeconomic Status and Preventive Health Behavior"; A. F. Williams and H. Wechsler, "Interrelationships of Preventive Actions in Health and Other Areas," *Health Services Reports*, vol. 87, December 1972, pp. 969–76; J. Steele and W. H. McBroom, "Conceptual and Empirical Dimensions of Health Behavior," *Journal of Health and Social Behavior*, vol. 13, December 1972, pp. 382–92; I. M. Rosenstock, "The Health Belief Model and Preventive Health Behavior," *Health Education Monographs*, vol. 2, Winter 1974, pp. 354–86;

32. Rosenstock, "Health Belief Model and Preventive Health Behavior,"; M. H. Becker, "Health Belief Model and Sick Role Behavior," *Health Education Monographs*, vol. 2, Winter 1974, pp. 409–19; S. V. Kasl, "The Health Belief Model and Behavior Related to Chronic Illness," *Health Education Monographs*, vol. 2, Winter 1974, pp. 433–54; J. H. Mitchell, "Compliance with Medical Regimens: An Annotated Bibliography," *Health Education Monographs*, vol. 2, Spring 1974, pp. 75–87.

33. Green, "Diffusion and Adoption of Innovations Related to Cardiovascular Risk Behavior in the Public"; Williams and Wechsler, "Interrelationships of Preventive Actions in Health and Other Areas"; Kasl, "Health Belief Model and Behavior Related to Chronic Illness"; L. W. Green, "Site- and Symptom-Related Factors in the Secondary Prevention of Cancer," in Bernard Fox, ed., "Applying Behavioral Sciences to Cancer Control" (Bethesda: National Cancer Institute, forthcoming).

Appendix M
The Prevention of Atherosclerotic Heart Disease:
An Example of the Political Context of Health Education and Behavior Change

by
Richard N. Podell, M.D., M.P.H.*

The Task Force's primary concern was the individual's health behavior and education. However, it was frequently necessary to enlarge this focus to include the political and social context in which the individual's health-related choices are being made. This is because of the profound influence the policies of government and other institutions may have on the individual's motivation and practical ability to choose a health-promoting life style or health-related alternative. For example, my ability and desire to exercise regularly is markedly inhibited since there are no bicycle lanes on the local roads and no bicycle paths in town. On the other hand, the availability of a restaurant near work which serves a variety of attractive salads and vegetarian dishes makes it easier to keep to a diet which will keep my cholesterol low.

During the course of discussion it became increasingly clear that many actions and policies which on the surface may seem unrelated to health actually have great influence on health-related choices, increasing the attractiveness of certain alternatives, and decreasing the value of others. The following outline of a national health strategy for the primary prevention of atherosclerotic heart disease illustrates the many-faceted, inevitably political, approach that has to be developed.

Heart disease was chosen to illustrate the point for several reasons: it is the leading cause of death among American adults; our heart disease death rates in middle age are double those in many other developed countries; a professional consensus is forming as to individual behaviors which could reduce heart disease, especially in the areas of cigarette smoking, diet, and hypertension. The outline is based on the report of the Inter-Society Commission for Heart Disease Resources.[1]

---

*Associate Director, Family Practice Training Program, Overlook Hospital, Summit, New Jersey; Consultant to CMDNJ-Office of Consumer Health Education; Member of Task Force on Consumer Health Education.

177

GENERAL RECOMMENDATIONS

A.   The President and Congress should recognize that a decrease in heart disease can be expected only if there is a reduction in heart disease risk factors. This in turn can occur only if more individuals choose a health-promoting life style. Therefore a cornerstone of national health policy should be to remove all obstacles to the individual's choices of health promoting behavior and to encourage individuals who request assistance in implementing such decisions and life style.

B.   The President and Congress should endorse as national health policy the goal of reducing cigarette smoking, cholesterol, and high blood pressure.

The President should appoint a panel chaired by the Secretary of Health Education and Welfare to review all government policy which inhibits the practical ability to fulfill these goals.

C.   In the development of plans for National Health Insurance, consideration should be given to mechanisms which would:

  1.   decrease the health insurance premium for individuals who do what is within their power to promote their own health;

  2.   scale payments to regional health institutions in part according to their actual record in reducing morbidity and mortality.

D.   The life insurance industry should use its influence to promote individual health, for example by offering financial incentive for applicants to stop smoking, control high blood pressure, and reduce elevated cholesterol.

E.   There should be established a National Center for Health Education and Promotion to encourage the research, evaluation, and demonstration of effective strategies of health education and preventive medicine.

F.   Third-party reimbursement should provide for the reimbursement for legitimate health education expenses. Health education and preventive procedures should be recognized and realistically emphasized under any proposal for National Health Insurance.

CIGARETTE SMOKING

A.   Since the elimination of cigarette smoking would have as great effect on reducing illness and premature death as any action now contemplated, this fact should be enunciated clearly by those formulating health policy.

B.   There should be a resumption of the national television advertising campaign to influence persons not to smoke.

C.   Recognizing the cigarette smoker is often psychologically and physiologically habituated to, and dependent on, cigarettes, as well as the expressed desire of many smokers to quit, and noting that scant funding is available for studies of the behavioral mechanisms of smoking cessation,

$10,000,000 should be allocated annually for such research. This would provide for laboratory research and also the community evaluation and demonstration of methods to prevent and to treat cigarette smoking.

D. In view of the potent pharmacological activity of the components of cigarette smoke, the Secretary of Health, Education, and Welfare together with the Food and Drug Administration should be empowered to establish maximum permissible levels for cigarettes of carbon monoxide, tars, and nicotine.

E. Recognizing the substantial interests of tobacco farmers and cigarette manufacturing companies, positive steps should be taken to promote their voluntary transfer of resources into other areas of economic activity. Subsidies for growing tobacco, however, are inconsistent with health priorities. Such subsidies should be abolished.

F. Public schools should routinely provide education on cigarette smoking. Funds should be alloted for the development and rigorous evaluation of such programs.

G. Federal law should mandate that 10 percent of income from cigarette taxes should be alloted to research, prevention, and treatment of diseases to which cigarette smoking contributes.

H. Continued support should be provided for the research and development of a safer cigarette.

FOOD AND NUTRITION

A. We note the opinion of the Council on Food and Nutrition of the American Medical Association and the Food and Nutrition Board of the National Academy of Sciences: "In summary, the average level of plasma lipids in most American men and women is undesirably elevated. . . . The evidence now available is sufficient to discourage further temporizing with this major national health problem."[2]

The prudent choice for most Americans is to:

1. reduce calorie intake and/or increase exercise to achieve ideal weight;
2. reduce daily cholesterol intake to less than 300 mg. per day;
3. reduce saturated fat intake to less than 10 percent of total calories.

B. The food industry is urged to adopt a policy which would:

1. provide the consumer with complete relevant nutrition information on all food products;
2. work toward removing legal and customary barriers to the development and sale of low-cholesterol, low-saturated fat foods;
3. increase research and development of attractive and economical substitutes for favorite high-saturated fat, high-cholesterol foods.

C.   The Food and Drug Administration should make mandatory the nutritional labeling of cholesterol and saturated fat content for foods high in cholesterol or saturated fat.

D.   The Federal Trade Commission should support the honest, aggressive, advertising of the low-saturated fat, low-cholesterol qualities of appropriate foods.

E.   The practical availability of low-cholesterol, and low-saturated fat food has been limited by hostile legislation and practices. In recent years there has been some progress.

The Filled Milk Act of 1928 has been declared unconstitutional. This Act forbade the passage in interstate commerce of milk in which milk fat was partly replaced by vegetable oil. Laws forbidding the sale of yellow margarine in certain states have been thrown out. Other laws and regulations prohibiting the sale of properly labeled meat and dairy products containing vegetable oil in place of meat or dairy fat have been repealed or rejected by the courts. However, substantial restrictions remain which artificially enhance the attractiveness of foods which are high in cholesterol and saturated fat:

1.   Mellorine is a form of ice cream in which milk fat can be partly replaced by unsaturated vegetable oil. Mellorine remains illegal in many states.

2.   Filled cheese is cheese in which some of the dairy fat has been replaced. Federal law provides that filled cheese may be sold only if the grocer pays a special tax and places a prominent sign stating "Filled Cheese Sold Here."

3.   Margarine is rarely available in restaurants. Skimmed milk often cannot be obtained. Attractive fruits, salad, fish, low-fat frozen desserts, low-saturated fat, and low-cholesterol baked goods are often difficult to find.

4.   In 1969 the federally funded school lunch program was found to provide an extraordinarily high proportion of fat calories as saturated fat. There has been some modification recently. Nevertheless, school lunch programs still provide a P/S ratio which is undesirably low. There is concern also as to the availability of low-cholesterol, low-saturated fat choices in government-sponsored cafeterias and other food programs.

5.   The Secretary of Agriculture is the government official with the most direct influence on national nutrition policy. In 1974 the Secretary of Agriculture urged Americans to eat more beef. He directed increased beef purchases for the school lunch program and other programs for which the federal government is responsible. No consideration was given to the health implication of adopting the promotion of beef consumption as government policy.

6.   Vending machines routinely promote foods which are high in satu-

rated fat and low in good nutrition. Low-saturated fat foods, such as fresh fruits, which are superior nutritionally from all points of view, are provided only rarely.

7. Restrictions remain on the degree to which high-quality vegetable protein imitation of meat may be offered in federal-government-sponsored food programs. Therefore we recommend:

a. Congress should declare null and void all laws and regulations which prohibit or discriminate against the manufacture or sale of any food solely because of its content of vegetable oil or vegetable protein. Regulation should instead be based on the actual nutritional quality. Clear and honest labeling should be required.

b. Government food programs and cafeteria menus and recipes should be required to provide attractive low-cholesterol, low-saturated fat meals for those desiring them.

c. Final responsibility for the nutritional content of the school lunch program should be transferred from the Department of Agriculture to the Department of Health, Education, and Welfare.

d. The President should appoint a committee to review all government programs and policies in the areas of food and nutrition to assess their compatibility with the principles of good nutrition and heart disease prevention. The Secretary of Health, Education, and Welfare should serve as chairman.

F. Many favorite foods are high in cholesterol and saturated fat. Many Americans have chosen substitutes for these foods which are nutritious, economical, and satisfying. Others find such alterations in their eating style to be a major burden. It is in the interest of the public health to encourage the food industry to develop more attractive substitutes for favorite high-cholesterol, high-saturated fat foods. Fully acceptable alternatives are technically feasible. The major obstacle is the expense of research, development, and marketing.

The federal government should provide tangible incentives for the food industry to develop attractive low-cholesterol, low-saturated fat foods, such as live stock with less fat and a lower proportion of saturated fat; eggs with lower cholesterol content; low-saturated fat versions of cheese, ice cream, and processed meats; baked goods and confectionaries low in cholesterol and saturated fat; cooking oils, salad dressings, and mayonnaise with less cholesterol and saturated fat.

The government should provide financial assistance to food manufacturers choosing to develop desirable new products in the form of research grants, contracts, and subsidy through the initial marketing phases.

G. Nutrition consultation should be provided under present third-party plans and under proposals for National Health Insurance.

H. Evaluation of serum cholesterol, along with other cardiovascular risk factors, should be performed routinely as part of the standard medical examination offered civilian and military government employees.

I. Nutrition education should be supported at all levels. Especially critical is the generally poor state of nutrition training for students in public schools and for public school teachers. Also important is support for the adequate training of professional nutritionists.

HYPERTENSION

A. We strongly support the policy of the federal government to view hypertension as a major health problem. We endorse current efforts to inform the public about hypertension and to identify individuals whose blood pressures are undesirably elevated.

However, more effort should be made to ensure that hypertension screening is effectively linked to appropriate treatment. The effectiveness of alternative approaches to high blood pressure detection, referral, and education should be evaluated. Particularly important is a better understanding of those elements promoting and inhibiting the patient's and the physician's ability and willingness to adhere to effective long-term hypertension management.

B. Medical Practice Acts in several states have been used to prevent allied health personnel from participating effectively in high blood pressure detection campaigns.

In our opinion, allied health workers such as pharmacists, optometrists, or trained nonprofessionals, *working within medically supervised guidelines in association with a medical treatment program,* should be encouraged to participate in high blood pressure identification.

C. Allied health personnel working from protocols have performed excellently in assisting the physician to monitor the maintenance treatment of a stable hypertensive patient. Regrettably, Medicare, Medicaid, and other third-party payers frequently will not reimburse for work done by such physician-supervised allied health workers. Reimbursement guidelines should be revised to encourage the use of physician assistants and physician extenders in appropriate clinical circumstances.

NOTES

1. *Circulation,* vol. 42, December 1970; the report was revised in April 1972.
2. The *Journal of the American Medical Association,* December 25, 1972.

Appendix N
Physician's Guide to Compliance in Hypertension

by
Richard N. Podell, M.D., M.P.H.*

INTERPRETIVE SUMMARY

Noncompliance occurs among persons of all social and economic classes, among all races and all personality types. The early literature on compliance seemed to assume that the "noncompliant patient" could be identified on the basis of sociodemographic or personality characteristics. In fact, the quest of unitary explanations based on the concept of the "noncompliant patient" has not succeeded and it should now be abandoned in favor of a more comprehensive approach. Several probable causes of noncompliant behavior have been discussed. Each makes a contribution, but none alone accounts for most of the behavior.

Health Education Strategies

Among the most useful approaches is that based on health education. Common sense suggests that better patient understanding should result in better compliance. Unfortunately, there has been no good test of this proposition to date. Indirect evidence suggests that the effect of general knowledge on compliance probably is modest at best. A much stronger case can be made for health education interventions which provide understanding of the *details* of particular treatment. In certain medical contexts, a substantial number of patients do not understand precisely what is expected of them after each visit. These patients have a much higher rate of noncompliance than patients who do understand. Therefore, a good case for *instructing patients more carefully* can be made.

Unfortunately, it is hard to distinguish between the effects of teaching the patient about his regimen and other closely associated effects. At the same time, the teacher almost invariably elicits feedback from the patient—for ex-

*Associate Director, Family Practice Training Program, Overlook Hospital, Summit, New Jersey; Consultant to CMDNJ-Office of Consumer Health Education; Member of Task Force on Consumer Health Education. Excerpted from Richard N. Podell, *Physician's Guide to Compliance in Hypertension*, 1975. Reprinted courtesy of Merck & Co., Inc.

ample, medication side effects, hidden noncompliance, fears, fantasies, questions, and covert patient priorities. This negative feedback may also result in compensatory action by the counselor. In addition, the fact that the counselor has shown interest in the patient's compliance might have some effect.

There is substantial evidence that each of these factors contributes to better compliance. Thus, patient education probably works through one or more of the following techniques: transmitting information about current treatment regimen and related concerns; eliciting negative feedback; applying specific motivating strategies; showing interest in the patient and in the patient's compliance. In practice, from the perspective of practical intervention, it may not be too important which method is most effective. Ordinarily, they may occur together with little or no more effort than would be required to apply one. McKenney's important study demonstrated a very dramatic increase in compliance from an ongoing health educational program which incorporated all four elements. One might also assume that if the *pharmacist* can effect such dramatic improvement in compliance, the *physician* can do as well or better.

What did the pharmacist do that the physician did not? Perhaps the difference was that the pharmacist deliberately set out to employ strategies that would increase patient compliance. In contrast, physicians are *less routinely aware* of the compliance issue and of the utility of health education. Svarstad demonstrated that some physicians use health education strategies frequently, while others do so rarely. We need to know what determines these choices and which of the strategies are the most important.

Adjusting the Therapeutic Regimen

A second approach which appears effective focuses on modifications in the actual therapeutic regimen. This approach overlaps the health education approach because of the importance of eliciting the patient's problems with the therapeutic regimen. The influence of medication side effects on noncompliance may remain hidden, especially if not asked about in detail.

Other adjustments in the therapeutic regimen are helpful. For some patients, *simplifying the regimen* will improve compliance. In selected individuals, a variety of aids will help the patient monitor himself better or improve convenience. For example, a pill box to carry the luncheon dose to work, a medication calendar, tying the dose in with daily habits such as brushing teeth, or enlisting family and social pressures to improve the supervision of medication-taking are all sometimes useful. In selected patients, modifying the therapeutic regimen may have dramatic effects on compliance.

The Patient's Health Beliefs

We have reviewed a number of sociological approaches which consider the patient's viewpoint of the doctor-patient relationship. Clearly, the health beliefs model and its close relatives account for part of the variability in patient compliance. The lesson is that the patient's *perception* of the whole situation is critical to cooperation. A patient must feel personally vulnerable to the sequelae of high blood pressure. He must perceive that the diagnosis is correct, that the treatment *is* useful, and that the doctor-patient relationship meets *his* perceived needs. Janis's work on fear, however, suggests that there is an *optimal level of perceived vulnerability*, beyond which compliance fails. In any case, what has been demonstrated is that it is the *patient's* interpretation of meaning which ultimately counts, not the doctor's.

A high priority for research should be an understanding of the development of health beliefs and an assessment of the degree to which these can be influenced.

To what degree are health attitudes and perceptions modifiable by current medical care contacts, educational material, or public relations campaigns? Our impression is that adult attitudes and perceptions do change, although seldom to the degree that we might wish to promote.[1,2]

Clinically, our best tack is to ask ourselves, "What are the patient's perceptions?" The asking of the question, by focusing on the patient rather than on the disease, may automatically lead to a more effective therapeutic stance.

All physicians employ motivating strategies sometimes; none employ them always. We do not know how the physician formulates strategy for each specific interaction. His compliance strategy would seem unplanned, almost accidental to an outsider. Few medical schools or residency programs take the problems of *communication with and motivating ambulatory patients* seriously enough to incorporate them in the formal curriculum. Most of us learn patient skills by trial and error *after* we are in practice. The evidence suggests that we might be more effective therapists if we would improve our ability to obtain compliance and if we deliberately trained ourselves in compliance-gaining techniques.

Doctor-Patient Interaction

The physician sets the tone of most medical interviews. He defines (and usually limits) the degree of patient participation, the degree of instruction, and the degree to which compliance-gaining strategies are used. Specific strategies include: giving explicit verbal and written instructions; monitoring for medication side effects; monitoring for noncompliance; explicitly justifying the therapeutic regimen; speaking of the regimens in tones of *positive* conviction and medical authority; indicating an openness to the patient's point of view and a willingness to entertain questions; telling the patient how he is doing; reinforcing the patient's sense of competence and good feeling about himself; eliciting and respecting the overt and covert issues on the patient's "agenda" which differ from those of the physician.

"Disease Denial and Rationalization"

The syndrome which we called "disease denial and rationalization" appears to be based on normal psychological processes, though often relatively exaggerated. By repeatedly becoming upset and protesting the request to pursue more aggressive therapy, the patient occasionally forces the physician into a kind of collusion. Doctor and patient quietly (even subconsciously at times) de-emphasize the goal of blood pressure control in the interest of maintaining harmony in the doctor-patient relationship.

We postulate that where patients are permitted more expression, the syndrome of "disease denial and rationalization" will be more common. Some cases of patient resistance are simply due to undeclared side effects from medications. Others occur with individuals whose priority concerns are not being addressed by the physician's *disease* orientation. Patient resistance may also derive from the physician's ambivalence as to the importance of pressing therapy once a moderate level of control has been obtained.

We are convinced that much patient resistance reflects genuine psychological defenses manifested to a greater than usual degree. Some patients cannot comfortably accept the diagnosis and treatment of high blood pressure. This may be because of the implied threat of death or disability, or the threat of self-image or social role. Who ever heard of a vigorous and youthful middle-aged sex symbol taking t.i.d. medication for high blood pressure? For other patients, the problem seems to be the loss of control, independence, and autonomy implied by the regular visits to the physician and daily taking of medication. For still others, there is a more specific aversion to drugs as a symbol of dependence and/or unnatural life-style. We suspect that the "disease denial and rationalization" syndrome is an important cause of poor blood pressure control. In some settings, it will manifest itself in a high dropout rate and covert noncompliance with pill-taking. In other settings, more open resistance and collusion to avoid conflict will also be seen. The challenge, of course, is *to obtain compliance without driving the patient away or sacrificing the therapeutic goal.*

Facilitating Compliance

We briefly considered the effect of improving the organization and structure of the medical setting. For most of us, immediate behavior is more motivated by current rewards and conveniences than by contemplation of possible future effects. Therefore, any actions which *make compliance more rewarding and more convenient now* should be of benefit. Finnerty has illustrated this better than anyone. He shortened the waiting time and created a clinic environment in which the patient is treated well. This, in conjunction with an outreach program, resulted in an impressive decrease in dropouts from 42% to 8%, which compared with the best in private practice.

A flow chart of hypertensive medications may limit the amount of time you need to spend during each visit reconstructing the patient's regimen. Give out printed cards with the date and time of the next appointment with you. Keep a follow-up file to note and pursue patients who don't show up for their high blood pressure check. *The attitudes of your staff are also important.* Most patients spend more time talking with the nurse than they do with you. Your staff must share your enthusiasm for treating high blood pressure and reinforce your concern with good compliance. Also, your staff may be an important source of negative feedback, which some patients are reluctant to give their physician.

Throughout this review of patient compliance, a recurring theme has been the crucial role of the *personal relationship* between the physician and patient. All the evidence suggests that patients do *not* view their physicians as interchangeable, the current practice in many hospital clinics notwithstanding. Substantial indirect evidence suggests that a continuous personal and individual doctor-patient relationship contributes importantly to better compliance.

NOTES

1. H. Leventhal, "Changing Attitudes and Habits to Reduce Risk Factors in Chronic Diseases," *American Journal of Cardiology*, vol. 31, 1973, p. 571.

2. S. T. Barnes and C. D. Jenkins, "Changing Personal and Social Behavior: Experiences of Health Workers in a Tribal Society," *Social Science Medicine*, vol. 6, 1972, p. 1.

Appendix O
Nutrition and Health

by
Barbara Echols Anlyan*

Diet, like smoking, is one of the few things affecting our general health and well-being over which we have a fair degree of control. Though our bodies are not in such "delicate balance" that we need constantly to monitor our food intake, there are certain groups more vulnerable to nutritional deficiencies than others: pregnant women, nursing mothers, infants, preschool children, adolescents, the poor, the elderly (especially those living alone), the chronically ill, and the sedentary.

One of the stumbling blocks to a better public understanding of the role that nutrition plays in health maintenance is the lack of a readily identifiable, reliable, national source for "state of the art" information. By and large, the public receives little help in dealing with controversial issues such as vitamin megadoses and dietary cholesterol. Rather, they must rely on the authority of whoever is presently in the news. Even weight control (one of our leading health problems) assistance is often hard to come by and, once again, the public is left to evaluate the safety of ketogenic diets, hypnotic suggestion, and a variety of shots and pills.

Traditionally, nutrition education has been offered as a part of home economics or has been tacked on to subjects such as biology or physical education. In many instances, nutrition education has not been offered in the schools at all. Even when available, nutrition education has consistently suffered from the major defect of lack of involvement of the intended audience in the planning of the program and, hence, lack of relevant subject matter and educational materials.

---

*Director, Office of Grants, Contracts, and Special Projects, Duke University Medical School, Durham, North Carolina; Author, "*Diet Is a 4-Letter Word*" (Barron's Educational Series, Inc., forthcoming); Nutrition consultant, North Carolina Department of Human Resources; Member of Task Force on Consumer Health Education.

As a consequence, we see programs focused on the three-meals-a-day, four-basic-food-groups patterns with little attention paid to individual preference and concerns, or ethical and economic considerations.

> Authoritative manuals abound on the need for vitamins and minerals and their importance in preventing scurvy, rickets, etc. But little is available to the general public citing both sides of the vitamin C megadose controversy.
> Vegetarianism is still often presented as "food fadism," and those concerned about food additives are viewed as "health food nuts."
> Dieters, like smokers, are told that "motivation" and "will power" are the answers to their dilemma. Little is offered in the way of linking knowledge to practical mechanisms that will enable people to adopt and maintain more healthful habits.

It is not surprising, then, that consumers exhibit a certain wariness when approached with additional information that is "good for them" to know.

VULNERABLE GROUPS AND HEALTH PROBLEMS RESPONSIVE TO NUTRITION INTERVENTION

Pregnancy Complications And Low Birth Weights

Nutritional deficiencies are most injurious during periods of rapid growth, such as in infancy, adolescence, and pregnancy. And pregnancy is the leading reason teenage girls leave school before graduation. Approximately 2 percent of all teenage births are to mothers *under* 15 years of age; this means 9,000–10,000 babies born to girls not yet grown themselves.

Births to teenage mothers comprise 17 percent of all births in the United States. The birth represents a first child for 77 percent of the teenagers, a second child for 18 percent, and a third or more child for 4 percent.

Late and irregular prenatal care is, unfortunately, characteristic of pregnant adolescents. Add to this lack of nutritional or any other guidance the emotional stress many of these youngsters face, and a sizable problem surfaces. Not only does the very young teenage mother run increased risks of complications of pregnancy, but the baby does not fare so well either. Premature delivery is not uncommon, and these babies face a greater chance of death or deformity than infants born to women at older ages.

Older teenage mothers do not seem to suffer unduly from pregnancy complications, but their babies still show lower birth weights than normal and increased risks of death or deformity. Whether or not the lower birth weights of children born to teenage mothers are attributable to the double nutritional stress of the mother's own adolescent growth plus that of her baby is not known. It has been claimed, however, that adolescent girls in the United States, regardless of socioeconomic status, usually have poorer diets than the rest of the members of a family.

Measures certainly need to be taken to improve the quality of prenatal care available for these girls, but even then it is probably unrealistic to expect a frightened and often very unhappy youngster to cope with the additional stress of a highly restricted or structured diet. A better approach is to begin sound nutrition education long before puberty to ensure the mother and the baby the safest pregnancy and delivery possible.

As would be expected, obese women have more problems during pregnancy than those of normal weight. However, markedly underweight mothers also have a higher incidence of preeclampsia than normal weight mothers.

The Nursing Mother

Anemia due to iron deficiency is common during and after pregnancy because of the large amount of iron given over to the fetus and enveloping placenta, the extra needs for increased red blood cell volume, and the large blood losses during delivery. A diet rich in iron is necessary, therefore, to protect the mother. It is also required so that the baby will be born with a liver well stored with iron to see him over the early months after birth when his diet will consist mainly of milk, a food low in iron content.

Even for a healthy woman with a good diet, the provision of enough milk to meet the needs of a vigorous infant is a physiological strain. When the mother's diet is inadequate, she will probably continue to supply milk, but her own stores of nutrients will be drawn upon, and evidence of maternal malnutrition may well appear.

This physiological stress is often compounded by the physical and emotional requirements of tending a new baby. The pale, chronically fatigued, new mother is an altogether too common sight. Continued concern for the mother's health is called for, in addition to postnatal guidance in the care of her infant.

Development During Infancy And The Early Years

The need for vitamins, minerals, and other nutrients for proper infant development is probably recognized, however vaguely, by most people. However, financial circumstances or incorrect knowledge about how to obtain these nutritional requirements or the serious consequences of their neglect deprives many a child of an adequate diet during this critical period of development when the body is growing more rapidly than at any other time during life.

The other extreme of nutrient neglect, poisoning, is also often seen. Vitamin poisoning is second only to aspirin poisoning in young children. This is occasionally the result of an overenthusiastic parent trying to "ensure" the child's health, but is more often the result of an accidental overdose.

The danger of excessive vitamin-mineral intakes is not widely known, and advertisements for super vitamins and vitamin-rich this, that, and the other do nothing to correct this. Perhaps unintentionally, many food and drug companies give the impression that if a little is good, a lot has to be better. And who can blame the child bombarded by this kind of message on television for scooping up a handful of vitamins made to look like chocolate-covered M&Ms?

Development During Adolescence

Growth in height proceeds more rapidly during the "adolescent growth spurt" than at any time since infancy. This, coupled with the increasing mobility and independence of the teenager, also makes this a time when radical changes in dietary practices are likely to occur. Vending machine offerings and "drive-in" foods play an increasing role in a teenager's life. This is also a time when there is great concern about body image, energy levels, and acne. At this point, teenagers are often receptive to concerned assistance in learning how to use food to better their physical appearance and abilities.

During adolescent growth, there are tremendous caloric and nutrient requirements. By and large these are met by regular meals augmented by snacking. The problem comes when the growth spurt has ceased, and consequently the need for so many calories. It is not uncommon for untoward weight gains to start at this time if the teenager doesn't make the necessary dietary cutbacks or doesn't exercise regularly. Actually, extreme physical inactivity seems to be more important as a root cause of obesity in children and adolescents than is overeating.

Great care must be taken in devising nutrition education programs at this stage, however, to make sure that the information provided is really relevant to the audience's perceived needs. A particularly common fault is to give too much information. Already many people are drowning in a sea of fragmentary facts about nutrition and food, without any real idea as to how the data relate to present problems, let alone future concerns.

Achievement For The Poor

Maslow, in describing the heirarchy of human needs, explains that the needs at one level must be reasonably satisfied before the need at the next level emerges and can be dealt with. The most basic human need relates to hunger and thirst. Assuring that every child has enough to eat has to precede any expectation for learning. Too often, however, school feeding is viewed as extraneous to education and is among the earlier programs to be considered for cutback when funds are short.

When extreme hunger is the normal condition, one cannot expect a positive approach to other aspects of living. Just as a hungry child cannot concentrate in school, the hungry adult cannot be a productive worker. If the cycle is not broken, the gap between the "haves" and the "have-nots" in a society will widen.

When looking at the dollars available to the poor, it is well to remember that a large percentage of the amount must go for food—especially at today's prices. Yet, ill-equipped kitchens, fatigue, and frequent ill health all combine to make the more expensive convenience foods even more important to the poor than to the prosperous.

One must also remember that the poor are exposed to the same inducements to buy as are all Americans, so that priorities are sometimes hard to set. The problems of the poor are complex, and they are not the same for all individuals. The poor are not a homogeneous group. They differ from each other psychologically, culturally, and ethnically, as well as in the degree of their poverty, the reasons for it, and the length of time it has been sustained.

The poor deserve respect for the many solutions to their own problems that they have evolved for themselves. Building on current practices is a more effective way to induce change than is criticism which is bound to arouse resentment.

Increasing The Quality Of Life For The Elderly And The Chronically Ill

Individuals over 65 years of age represent almost 10 percent of the population of the United States—approximately 20 million people. This age group is increasing in numbers more rapidly than is the population at large, and census experts predict that by the year 2000 at least 30 million people in the United State will be 65 or older—and this is assuming that significant breakthroughs in the treatment and prevention of cancer and cardiovascular-renal diseases do not occur!

One of the major problems of the elderly with regard to obtaining an adequate diet is low income. The poor and the elderly represent widely overlapping groups in our population. Another problem relates to chronic illness. It is estimated that three-fourths of the noninstitutional population over 65 have one or more chronic conditions, and that almost 2 out of 5 have a chronic condition that limits their activity.

The fact that caloric needs decrease with age due to reduced basal metabolic rate and reduced physical activity, without proportional decreases in the needs for protein, vitamins, and minerals, may make the elderly person vulnerable to nutrient deficiency. Additionally, as people grow older they may lose the motivation to apply the knowledge that they already have, and attempts to improve nutrition must include efforts to improve the individual's desire to help himself as well as to provide accurate nutrition information.

There are increasing efforts to improve the quality of the older person's life rather than just aiming for longevity. Early preventive nutritional practices may help ward off some of the problems of illness associated with heart and other diseases, but continuing good nutrition should also be a part of the campaign.

Problems Of The Sedentary

The American life style has become more and more sedentary as prosperity and labor-saving devices have reduced the amount of manual labor required to earn a living and maintain a home. Along with these "advances" has come an increased incidence of heart disease and obesity.

Heart disease continues to be the leading cause of death in the United States. There are a number of different kinds of heart disease, but almost all are associated with atherosclerosis, a degenerative condition in which the arteries thicken, the space in the artery is narrowed, and the arteries become less elastic. It is disturbing that autopsies done on very young children who died from accidents, etc., show the beginnings of some of these disease processes which may have claimed their lives in later years had they survived infancy. Autopsies done on young soldiers in their twenties revealed a large amount of hardening of the arteries.

Obesity not only aggravates cardiovascular diseases but also increases the likelihood of their development. Excessive weight overworks even a normal heart and circulatory system, let alone a damaged one. Add to this physical strain the excessive amounts of fat eaten and stored and the reduced exercise pattern of most obese people, and you have a blueprint for disaster.

From various statistical data, we can draw a picture of the coronary-prone individual. He is a middle-aged male, markedly overweight, has a history of heart disease in his family, and has high blood pressure and elevated cholesterol and triglyceride levels. He smokes more than a pack of cigarettes a day, is hardworking but holds a job requiring little physical exertion, and habitually eats food high in saturated fats and cholesterol.

It is interesting that strenuous physical exercise seems to protect against coronary heart disease, even in the presence of a diet which is typical of those found in populations where the incidence of atherosclerosis is high. Also, other studies have shown that people in physically active jobs have less coronary heart disease, and that even when they do develop heart disease it is less severe and appears later in life than in people with physically inactive jobs.

Though heart transplantation or mechanical hearts may be possible in this day of scientific miracles, it is not possible to replace all the blood vessels that can get plugged up and lead to heart disease. Prevention is the answer.

Obesity And The Child

Most physicians agree that obesity is one of our leading health problems today. What many people do not realize is the large number of adolescents who are overfat and the consequences of this. It is estimated that at least 10 million preadults are carrying around unhealthy fat. Couple this figure with statistics that clearly show that extreme overweight shortens one's lifespan, increases the incidence of heart disease, gall bladder disease, and diabetes, and increases the dangers of complications of pregnancy and surgery and the likelihood of accidents due to slowed reflexes—not to mention the tremendous psychological cost—and a health problem of staggering proportions emerges.

The more excessive the overweight and the older the person, the greater the likelihood of suffering from the health hazards associated with overweight. Unfortunately, however, it is well documented that obese children run a great risk of remaining obese all their lives. It has been estimated that for obese children of age 12, the odds against being normal-weight adults are 4 to 1, and if weight loss is not accomplished by the end of adolescence, the odds rise to 28 to 1.

The obese child presents special and difficult problems, for treating the obese child involves treating the parents as well, since they control the eating and exercise patterns of children to a great extent. The magnitude of the obesity problem in youngsters is such that reliance cannot be placed on the individual initiative of parents and children to obtain weight therapy when needed. Furthermore, the cost of such therapy through private medicine is generally too high for all but a limited number of individuals. The public school system, therefore, affords one suitable and logical focus for an attack on the problem of weight control,

Food and eating should remain a pleasure for both parent and child, but it should also be remembered that the framework for lifetime eating patterns is well established before the child enters school. Many habits and attitudes are good and are intentionally fostered by parents, but some are bad and are unintentionally determined. For example, consider the effect of withholding dessert as a form of punishment for bad behavior or using it as a reward for "cleaning your plate"; either way, dessert is likely to assume undue importance. Likewise, using a bottle or other food as a pacifier to distract a fretful child may well set the stage for the development of a pattern of eating when bored or under stress.

Our educational system doesn't prepare young men and women for the care and feeding of infants, and new parents must rely heavily on the advice of their own parents or others. Unfortunately, many nutritional myths are perpetuated this way. Then, too, physician advice ("Feed the baby four ounces of milk *every* four hours") is often followed too literally, and the result is an overfed child. Greater care in prescribing dietary regimes and assessing family understanding seems warranted.

Vegetarianism

A number of our young people are avoiding meat for a variety of reasons and are, or probably will be, rearing their children in like fashion. By and large, vegetarians are a healthy lot, suffering from nutritional deficiencies no more than most of us. If, however, milk and egg products are also avoided, great care is called for to avoid vitamin B12, iron, zinc, and calcium deficiencies. The biggest problem, however, is to obtain all the essential amino acids, especially during growth periods. This requires a careful balancing of food as all of the essential amino acids must be present at the same meal for any one of them to do its proper job.

Nutritional deficiencies are harmful to all, but they are especially dangerous when the body is in a growth period. A small but significant number of cases with severe deficiencies have already been reported where milk and egg products have been excluded from the diet. If irreversible damage to the child's health and body is to be avoided, we must provide the necessary dietary information required to provide an adequate diet without unduly compromising the parents' dietary beliefs. Otherwise, their offspring may be lost to medical surveillance for ever.

Dental Health For Everyone

Our nation's dental bill is staggering—over 4 billion dollars a year—yet it is estimated that 1 out of every 5 Americans will need dentures by the age of 45. Early attention to preventive measures is necessary if we are to reverse this trend.

The life of a tooth begins long before birth, while the baby is still being formed. Successful tooth development is, therefore, initially dependent on the adequacy of the mother's nutrition. For the continuation of tooth formation after birth, the baby must still rely on the mother to provide the proper nutrients, either from her own body stores by way of breast feeding or by "formula" supplementation.

In this country, dental ill health is probably related more to faulty eating habits and inadequate oral hygiene than to poor nutrition. Sticky carbohydrates such as white bread and candy, when not removed promptly from the teeth, provide an excellent breeding ground for the bacteria to start the work that leads to cavities. Diets consisting largely of soft foods, combined with inadequate brushing of the teeth, allow tartar to accumulate at a surprising rate, and often lead to serious periodontal disease.

Fluorine plays an important role in preventing tooth decay and, hence, in most parts of this country this element is added to our public water supply. Some localities have no need of fluorine addition as their water already contains adequate amounts of this mineral. Yet other areas have the problem of an excess of fluorine occurring naturally in their water supply, which results in teeth resistant to dental decay but which also produces an unattractive brown-stained enamel.

There is still much public confusion about the various factors involved in tooth decay and its prevention. Many fears about fluoridation are based on scanty and incorrect knowledge. There is still much need for public education.

Another need is for companies and agencies providing prepaid medical insurance plans to extend their coverage to include routine dental examinations and treatment. And it is imperative that we do something about providing free dental care for families with reduced incomes. It makes no sense to provide free meals if the children aren't going to have any teeth with which to eat them.

POSSIBLE APPROACHES TO BETTER NUTRITION

The fundamental philosophy of nutrition education is that prevention is preferable to cure. In terms of money, time, quality of life, and human resources, it can be shown repeatedly that rehabilitation is more costly than prevention. Efforts to focus on prevention of nutritional ill health rather than solely on crisis intervention are needed.

Each group in the previous section represents a complex series of problems, with nutrition being but one of the many elements involved. In each situation, however, it is possible that improving the state of nutrition may also benefit the other problem areas; the reverse is, of course, also true.

Common to all the problems discussed earlier is the need to influence the developing food and exercise habits of the young child. Additionally, programs are needed to educate the public better regarding the availability of prenatal clinics and other health services, their right and need to use these facilities, and *how* to use them effectively. Also, the public and their elected representatives need a clearer picture of the nutritional needs of the country—health and health insurance providers, public assistance programs, and the food industry all have responsible roles and should stand accountable. Nor can we forego our worldwide responsibilities. Cattle being slaughtered and discarded while people starve to death shows a recklessness and lack of concern for human life and suffering that is hard to comprehend. One of the consequences of our affluence is a lack of appreciation for just how precious food is to many people.

Specific educational efforts might include the following:

1. Support of legislation aimed at increasing the number of professionals qualified to teach comprehensive health education at the elementary and secondary school level.

2. Development of funding sources for pilot and demonstration projects to reassess health education goals and the relevance of current teaching material and practices to present and future needs of elementary-and secondary-

school students, and for curriculum and materials development and dissemination.

3. Initiation of school-based programs aimed at weight evaluation and regulation. Cooperation from the medical community and parents would be necessary to assess safely the individual's health and the advisability of participating in such an endeavor. The presence of such a project might make both physicians and parents more alert and sympathetic to the minimally overweight person rather than waiting until they're markedly overweight. An extra few pounds is more easily and more satisfactorily dealt with than the burden of twenty or thirty pounds and their attendant illnesses. Preventive rather than curative medicine is advocated for other areas of bodily concern —why not for fat control?

4. As the character of the available food supply changes to include increasing reliance on fabricated foods, vending machines, and out-of-home feeding in general, nutrition education efforts directed toward food suppliers are increasingly important. What is available at school, at work, and in the local drive-in will influence the quality of our diet. The individuals who decide what vending machines to install in a factory or a school, for instance, are important targets of nutrition education.

5. A tremendous amount of money is being spent by food manufacturers for the promotion of their products. Considering the influence that the advertising media has over the public's eating habits; if even a part of this effort were directed at reorienting Americans' tastes, it would be a great contribution to the nation's health. It is hoped that the food industry and television broadcasting companies will become increasingly concerned about their public role and responsibilities.

6. Federal regulations require labels to indicate nutritional composition if the foods are "enriched" or "fortified" or if a nutritional claim is made for the food. Other foods are not required to be so labeled. Many companies have started voluntarily including this type of information on their products' labels. This trend indicates a definite concern for the health of the American people and should be applauded and further encouraged. An educational program will, however, be required if the public is to understand and make use of this information.

7. It is impractical to expect individual restaurants to change their preparation practices or at least to post the caloric values of their foods, but it is not untoward to expect this of school and office cafeterias. There is much that still isn't known about nutritional needs and the consequences of certain deficiencies and excesses, but that which *is* known shouldn't be so blatantly disregarded by institutions responsible for feeding large segments of our society—especially our children. People deserve sufficient information to know what nutrient choices they are making.

8. Exercise not only helps ward off obesity but it helps to keep arteries unclogged and increases chances of recovery in the event of a heart attack. Unfortunately, however, Americans seem to have not only trouble motivating themselves to exercise, but difficulty in motivating their children as well. By the time the average child starts school, he has logged over 4,000 hours in front of the television set! To compound the issue, most physical education programs at school and in the community are aimed at the person who is already in good physical condition. Increased opportunities are needed for obese or otherwise handicapped people to improve their physical activity pattern. Also, patterns of more individual exercise should be encouraged if a life-long pattern of participation is to be encouraged. A tennis partner is easier to locate than enough people for a football or volleyball game.

9. To improve the nutrition of the elderly, and to take advantage of the influence they exert over younger members in the family, every effort should be made to update their nutritional information. Again, the data provided need to be relevant to their needs. Community programs for the elderly and various hobby clubs are two modes of approach. Contacts with club members representing a younger age group might also get the message carried home to parents and grandparents. Businesses could also probably be persuaded to offer preretirement seminars and discussions for their employees, provided adequate instructional materials and guidance were available.

10. Continued research into the relationship of nutrition to health and illness needs to be conducted. In many cases, this may require stimulating faculty to an awareness and interest in the area. Few medical schools have an organizational cluster identified with nutritional concerns. One obvious problem here is the lack of manpower trained or knowledgeable in the field. New types of training experiences may well be called for.

11. Professionals active in the field of nutrition must take increased responsibility for educating the public at large about their perceived needs and concerns. The number of food-related books that are in print and are being purchased clearly attests to the public's concern with diet. Much of the information published is, without question, incorrect or misleading. Too often, however, knowledgeable people and organizations merely attack these lay-oriented publications without offering practical advice in their stead. It is little wonder, then, that the public often views health-related professionals as being in an adversary position and turn instead to the miracle-offerers.

12. Hospitals and long-term care facilities offer another possibility for educating the public about nutritional concerns. To be effective, however, the food in these institutions would probably have to become more palatable and more responsive to the needs of the individual. Serving the same caloric offering to the 100 and 250 pounder alike doesn't say much for the hospitals' awareness of individual needs.

This material is intended to provide a brief introduction to the role that nutrition can play in maintaining one's health. An in-depth or comprehensive discussion has not been the intent. And though reimbursement and evaluation mechanisms have not been dealt with, their omission should not be construed as indifference to the problems. By the same token, the difficulties involved in financing and assessing health education endeavors should not keep us from trying to move on with the resources at hand.

Appendix P
Financial Incentives as an Aid to
Health Education

by
Mary Ashley*

This is to present some of my own thinking on the use of monetary reinforcers as incentives for desired behaviors. Our present system of government and our personal value systems are greatly influenced by incentives. A man's worth is often measured by how much money he has or earns. Money is one of the greatest reinforcers in our culture.

I am, therefore, suggesting that a viable system of monetary incentives for both providers and consumers be initiated in this country. It could be administered in the form of tax breaks. For example, physicians who practice in high risk urban areas should receive extra incentives. Each person who presents evidence of a physical and dental examination within a year would get a tax break—for example, a $100 deduction. Those who had corrective therapy for any condition would get a $125 deduction. Children between one and ten years who are completely immunized would receive a tax credit. The provider would get tax credit for each person he sees on successive years for preventive, but not corrective, therapy. I am sure there are many individuals who develop a creative, feasible approach to tax incentives, which are used widely in other areas of our economy.

I am convinced that changes in behavior will not occur in either providers or consumers until it is more profitable to engage in new behaviors than it is to maintain their old patterns.

*Coordinator of Health Education, Department of Community Medicine, Charles R. Drew Postgraduate Medical School, Los Angeles, California; Member of Task Force on Consumer Health Education.

Appendix Q
Assistant Secretary for Health:
Statement of Functions*

Public Health Service

THE ASSISTANT SECRETARY FOR HEALTH

Statement of Organization, Functions, and Delegations of Authority

Part 1 of the Statement of Organization, Functions, and Delegations of Authority for the Department of Health, Education, and Welfare, Office of the Secretary is amended to delete Chapter 1N, Office of the Assistant Secretary for Health, (38 FR 18571, July 12, 1973, as amended), which is renumbered and superseded by new Chapter 15, The Assistant Secretary for Health. The new Chapter reads as follows:

Section 15-A Mission. The Assistant Secretary for Health is responsible for the direction of the Public Health Service, for providing leadership and policy guidance for health-related activities throughout the Department and for maintaining relationships with other governmental and private agencies concerned with health. The Assistant Secretary for Health is the principal advisor and assistant to the Secretary on health policy and all health-related activities in the Department.

Section 15-B Organization. The Assistant Secretary for Health directs the activities of the Public Health Service, which is composed of the following:

Office of the Assistant Secretary for Health
Alcohol, Drug Abuse, and Mental Health Administration
Center for Disease Control
Food and Drug Administration
Health Resources Administration
Health Services Administration
National Institutes of Health
Public Health Service (PHS) Regional Offices

Federal Register, August 20, 1974.

Section 15-C Functions. A. Office of the Assistant Secretary for Health. 1. Assistant Secretary for Health. Provides leadership and guidance on all health and health-related activities, including research and development; education and training; organization financing and delivery of health care services; and problems of public and environmental health. In addition, he is responsible for the direction of nursing home affairs throughout the Department; and exercising specialized responsibilities in the areas of population affairs, international health, and transportation and disposition of certain hazardous materials. He coordinates the health and health-related functions of the Department with those of other Federal agencies and provides advice and assistance on health matters to such agencies as requested.

That part of Chapter 1N beginning with the heading "Executive Secretariat" is incorporated within the new Chapter 15 following Section 15-C.

Dated: August 12, 1974.

CASPAR W. WEINBERGER.

Secretary.

Appendix R
Department of Health, Education, and Welfare
Public Health Service

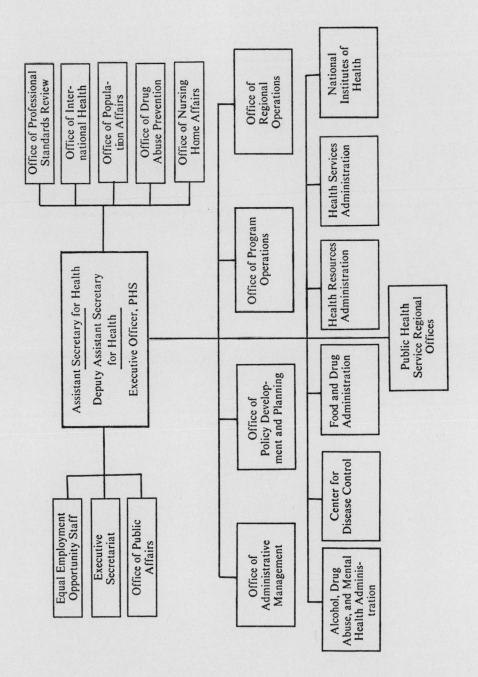

Appendix S
Bureau of Health Education:
Statement of Functions*

Public Health Service

CENTER FOR DISEASE CONTROL

Statement of Organization, Functions, and Delegations of Authority

Part 9 (Center for Disease Control) of the Statement of Organization, Functions, and Delegations of Authority for the Department of Health, Education, and Welfare (39 FR 1461, January 9, 1974) is hereby amended to reflect the establishment of the Bureau of Health Education (9F00) and the transfer of the National Clearinghouse for Smoking and Health (9S00) to the Bureau of Health Education as indicated in the following changes to Section 9-B, *Organization and Functions:*

1. After the chapter entitled "Bureau of Epidemiology (9E00)," add a new chapter entitled "Bureau of Health Education (9F00)" by inserting the following heading and succeeding paragraphs:

BUREAU OF HEALTH EDUCATION (9F00)

(1) Provides leadership and direction to a comprehensive national health education program for the prevention of disease, disability, premature death, and undesirable and unnecessary health problems; (2) recommends health education goals, objectives, and priorities for the Department of Health, Education, and Welfare; and develops collaborative efforts to accomplish health education objectives; (3) coordinates major health education activities of the Department; (4) develops and evaluates standards, criteria, and methodologies for improved health education programs; (5) serves as a clearinghouse on health education; (6) working with and through the

---

Federal Register, September 24, 1974.

Regional Offices, encourages and assists in the broader application of effective health education programs at the State and community level; (7) develops mechanisms for coordinating health education activities of the private sector; (8) participates in, and provides staff support for, the Intradepartmental Health Education Board; (9) provides leadership and direction for a national program to reduce death and disability due to smoking; (10) maintains liaison with other Federal agencies and with public and private organizations engaged in health education activities.

Office of the Director (9F01). (1) Plans, directs, coordinates, and evaluates activities of the Bureau; (2) provides leadership and guidance in policy formulation and program planning and development; (3) participates in, and provides staff support for, the Intradepartmental Health Education Board; (4) develops mechanisms for coordinating health education activities of the private sector; (5) provides consultation and assistance to CDC organizations in developing and implementing health education activities; (6) maintains liaison with other Federal agencies engaged in health education activities; (7) provides overall administrative services to the Bureau.

National Clearinghouse for Smoking and Health (9F41). (1) Administers a national program to reduce death and disability due to smoking; (2) develops standards, criteria, and methodologies for improved health education programs; and evaluates effectiveness of selected ongoing programs; (3) serves as a clearinghouse on health education; collects and disseminates information about effective techniques, strategies, and approaches; and handles health education inquiries; (4) conducts and stimulates behavioral research; (5) coordinates Department activities related to smoking and health, and maintains liaison with official and voluntary groups concerned with the problem of smoking; (6) conducts surveys to assess the incidence of smoking.

Community Program Development Division (9F45). (1) Develops, conducts, and evaluates health education demonstration projects, in cooperation with State and local health departments and with public and private organizations, to develop and apply effective, comprehensive programs in selected communities; (2) develops and applies new combinations of approaches and methods to unmet public health education needs.

Professional Services and Consultation Division (9F49). (1) Provides technical advice and consultation to State and local health agencies, and to public and private organizations in planning and implementing health education activities; (2) working with and through the Regional Offices, encourages and assists in the broader application of effective health education programs at the State and community level; (3) assists the Office of the Bureau Director in coordinating health education activities of the private sector.

2. Delete the chapter entitled "National Clearinghouse for Smoking and Health (9S00)."

Dated: September 16, 1974.

JOHN OTTINA,
*Assistant Secretary for
Administration and Management.*

Appendix T
National Health Education and
Promotion Act of 1975

Hon. Tim Lee Carter
of Kentucky

IN THE HOUSE OF REPRESENTATIVES
Thursday, April 10, 1975

MR. CARTER. Mr. Speaker, when we consider the cluster of concerns that we commonly call our national health care crisis, we usually look to megaproposals which demand great expenditures of funds and major systems revisions, or to proposals that are so financially modest and lacking in substance as to be meaningless.

We find ourselves today struggling with various efforts at reorganization, rationalization, and regulation of health services, seeking improvements in financing mechanisms, pondering the problems associated with health manpower, and invariably ending up considering derivative proposals, or proposals which are variations of themes dating to the first decade of this century, as if they were bold, new, and imaginative.

We have sold our society on the wonders of modern medicine and we have created an insatiable demand for services. Only recently, Mr. Speaker, have we recognized that there are limits to the amount and kind of resources that we can allocate to health care.

We find ourselves with only a few possibilities. We can reduce demand by reinstating financial barriers to access, by imposing monetary limits on prices or overall expenditures, or by rationing available resources.

Mr. Speaker, we no longer have the option of unlimited spending for personal health services, and yet I do not believe that the American people will accept the reimposition of financial barriers as a legitimate way of controlling demand. Therefore, I am introducing a proposal that offers the alternative strategy of health education and health promotion.

213

I am also introducing this health education proposal to prod our collective memories. It seems that somehow we have forgotten, perhaps because we have been unduly and overly impressed by the sophistication and technology of modern medicine, that mechanisms for the delivery of health care are only one of the many ways of maintaining and improving health. Let me recall for you that, although much of our health progress stems from remarkable advances in scientific medicine of the last and early part of the present century and their applications in the prevention and treatment of disease, our improved health status also reflects in considerable degree the improvements in general living conditions and improved sanitary measures as well. Better housing, nutrition, working conditions, and education enhance the health of our people just as certainly as better health services.

It is reassuring, then, to note the recent rekindling of interest in consumer health education, health promotion and preventive medicine. For example, mention was made in former President Nixon's health message of the need to moderate self-imposed risks and of the realization that each of us bears the major responsibility for our health. There has been a President's Committee on Health Education; Blue Cross and the American Hospital Association have endorsed the concept of patient health education; and, HEW's forward plan presents prevention as its first, major health planning theme. Also, the new National Health Planning and Resources Development Act considers prevention and health education national health priorities as do the statutes creating health maintenance organizations, while in Canada, the Minister of Health and Welfare has produced a remarkable document which presents a new health promotion perspective which will be embodied in future Canadian health programs.

This interest in health education activities is not without a rationale. Health care costs have risen at an alarming rate. The data indicate that inflation of health care costs has occurred at a rate considerably in excess of the Nation's general inflation. Despite our huge outlays in dollars and resources our health indicators reveal that we are obviously not getting our money's worth. We have more physicians per capita than any other country in Europe or North America and yet, at each age from infancy through middle age and into the seventies, the rate of death of Americans is almost the highest in the developed world.

Why then have we gained so little health benefit from our tremendous investment in health services? Certainly, for a part of America the reason is lack of access to medical care of high quality, but for the majority of Americans the answer lies in the changing nature of disease. It is now the chronic diseases and the diseases of advanced civilization and changing lifestyles that concern us.

The principal causes of death in our country are owing to motor vehicle accidents, ischaemic heart disease, other accidents, respiratory diseases and lung cancer, and suicide. Please note, Mr. Speaker, that self-imposed risks and environmental factors are the principal or important underlying factors in each of the five major causes of death betweeen the age of 1 and age 70. It is a safe conclusion that unless lifestyles and self-imposed risks are modified or the environment changed, the death rates will not be significantly improved.

If we momentarily review morbidity rates as collated from a study of illness requiring hospitalization, we have further proof of changing disease patterns. Diseases of the cardiovascular system are the principal cause of hospitalization. Fractures and head injuries, burns and all other causes arising from accidents or violence follow in scale. For such causes of hospitalization, individual behavior and carelessness are the principal or important underlying factors.

From Marc Lalonde's Canadian working document there appears this interesting litany, indicating some of our more destructive lifestyle habits and their consequences. For example, alcohol addiction, he writes, leads to cirrosis of the liver, encephalopathy and malnutrition; abusing pharmaceuticals leads to drug dependence and drug reactions; addiction to psychotropic drugs leads to suicide, homicide, malnutrition, and accidents; overeating leads to obesity; highfat intake possibly contributes to atherosclerosis and coronary artery disease; high carbohydrate intake contributes to dental caries; lack of recreation and lack of relief from other pressures are associated with stress diseases such as hypertension, coronary-artery disease and peptic ulcer; promiscuity leads to venereal disease; and careless driving, and failure to wear seatbelts, leads to accidents and resultant deaths and injuries.

If we turn to the social and physical environment, about which individuals can do little, we find that public health and governmental application is both imperfect and uneven. I speak of air, water and noise pollution and the failure of many communities to fluoridate their drinking water. Also, urbanization, crowding, adverse working conditions, and rapid social change all effect mental and physical health in ways we do not yet fully understand.

When you take such factors into consideration, Mr. Speaker, you may agree that health status cannot be equated with the organization, financing and delivery of health services alone. Outstanding though our health services are, there is no doubt that if we are to improve our level of health we must turn to a new strategy, one which will assist us to understand the nature and causes of self-imposed risks, adds to our knowledge of illness, educates patients and consumers about health maintenance and prevention, and improves the physical and social environment.

Let me pursue this point about patient education further. Consider the treatment for diabetes mellitus. What are the respective roles for the doctor and the patient? Ideally the disease should be discovered early. The physician makes a diagnosis and prescribes therapy. The patient must inject himself with the correct dosage of insulin every day, interpret his own urine samples and decide when a change is sufficient to warrant calling his physician. The patient must be motivated to lose weight, recognize and report side effects, learn proper techniques for foot and toenail care to avoid the devastating complication of infection and gangrene, recognize early symptons of complications, and visit his physician when scheduled. The physician's role is essential to effective treatment; so too is the patient's. No amount of resources devoted to physician or hospital care can substantially reduce the cost of diabetes if the patient has not been adequately trained and motivated to do his part.

When such a patient education program is well thought out it has proved to be very successful. In the Los Angeles County Medical Center diabetes education program, a telephone "hotline" was introduced for information, medical advice, and for obtaining prescription refills. Patients were educated to use this service through an aggressive campaign of pamphlets, posters, and counseling sessions by physicians and nurses. When the program was evaluated, it was found that the incidence of diabetic coma was reduced from 300 to 100, the number of emergency visits by the diabetic patients were reduced by half, and that 2,300 clinic visits were avoided. Over 2 years, total savings was estimated at more than $1.7 million.

Similar positive results were found with patient education programs for asthma, congestive heart failure, hypertension, hemophilia, and pain following surgery. But such physician and hospital initiatives are limited owing to lack of funds. Furthermore, we do not at this time understand fully the nature of health motivation and how individuals chose between health promoting and illness promoting behavior. We need more research; we need careful evaluation of health education programs to determine which are effective and which are not; and, we need to recognize that Government itself often inadvertently works to promote individual habits and exposures which promote disease.

So, Mr. Speaker, we have had presidential messages, task force and commission reports and the occasional statute and authorization for consumer health education programs. There is even a Bureau of Health Education in the Center for Disease Control in Atlanta, Ga., although very few know of this fact. But despite the study commissions and the activity in both the public and private sectors there is still no national program or adequate central force to stimulate and coordinate a comprehensive health education program. Our efforts are fragmented. The moneys we spend for health education, health promotion, and preventive medicine are miniscule. There is no informational exchange between those public and private agencies and organizations concerned with health education; there has been little evaluation of results among similar or related health education programs sponsored by different organizations; information about health education theory, programs and methods is not easily accessible; there is presently no agency, public or private, which is systematically reviewing the broad range of experience and theoretical experimentation in health education and related fields; and, there is no focal point to facilitate communication and cooperation among the significant health organizations in and out of Government which must work together if substantial improvement in health education is to be achieved.

Mr. Speaker, the needs, problems, and opportunities are so large, urgent, and complex that progress will depend upon a major long-term commitment by both the public and private sectors of society. To meld such efforts, provide a focal point for the Nation's multiple but disparate health education activities, improve the health status of Americans, design a mechanism by which we may establish a national health education, health promotion and preventive medicine strategy, I am now submitting for congressional action the National Health Education and Promotion Act of 1975.

I include a section-by-section analysis of my bill in the Record:

Section 1 states that the title of the Act is the National Health Education and Promotion Act of 1975.

Title I. National Center for Health
Education and Promotion

Section 101 establishes the National Center for Health Education and Promotion within the Department of Health, Education and Welfare and declares that the Center shall be supervised by the Department's principal health officer and shall be organized with no less than the following four divisions:

(a) Research in health education and preventive medicine,

(b) Community health education programs,

(c) Communications in health education and,

(d) Federal programs.

Section 102 provides that the Secretary shall:

(1) formulate a national strategy and national goals with respect to health education, health promotion, and preventive medicine;

(2) develop an integrated and comprehensive perspective on national health education, health promotion, and preventive medicine needs and resources, and recommend appropriate educational and certifying policies for health education and preventive medicine manpower;

(3) incorporate appropriate health education components into every facet of our society, especially into all aspects of health care and educational programming;

(4) increase the application of health knowledge, skills, and practices by the general population in their patterns of daily living;

(5)   increase the effectiveness and efficiency of health education and preventive medicine programs through improved planning, implementation of tested models, and evaluation of results;

(6)   establish systematic processes for the exploration, development, demonstration, and evaluation of innovative health education concepts; and

(7)   foster information exchanges and cooperation among health education providers, consumers, and supporters.

The Section also provides that the Secretary shall carry out this Title consistent with Title XV of the Public Health Service Act, which relates to health planning and development.

Section 103 (a) provides that the Secretary, through the division of research in health education and preventive medicine, shall conduct and support research in health education, health promotion, and preventive medicine.

This Section also provides that the National Center for Health Statistics, which is established under Section 306 of the Public Health Service Act, shall make continuing surveys of the needs, interests, attitudes, knowledge, and behavior of the American public regarding health. The Secretary shall use the findings of these surveys together with the findings of surveys conducted by other organizations in formulating policy respecting health education and promotion, and preventive medicine. This section authorizes appropriations of $3,000,000 for fiscal year 1976, $4,000,000 for 1977, and $5,-000,000 for 1978 for activities of the National Center for Health Statistics.

Section 103 (b) (1) provides that the Secretary, acting through the division of community health education programs, shall support and encourage new and innovative programs in health education and preventive medicine.

Section 103 (b) (2) provides that the Secretary may not approve any application of any health care facility for a grant under the Public Health Services Act or the Community Mental Health Centers Act in any fiscal year beginning after the passage of this act unless the facility includes consumer health education programs prescribed through regulations by the Secretary of Health, Education, and Welfare.

Section 103 (b) (2) also provides that the consumer health education services must be offered by health care providers as a condition of eligibility for payments under Title XVIII of the Social Security Act and that the Secretary should enter into agreements with the States under which the States would require health care providers within their jurisdictions to provide consumer health education as a condition of payment under Title XIX of the Social Security Act. This provision would take effect in the calendar quarter beginning more than 90 days after the passage of this Act.

Section 103 (c) provides that the Secretary, acting through the division of communications in health education shall establish liaison between the Center and providers of health education services and the communications media.

Section 103 (d) provides that the Secretary, acting through the division of Federal programs shall:

(1) make recommendations to the Congress for the inclusion in appropriate legislation of provisions respecting health education and promotion;

(2) establish a liaison with other Federal agencies engaged in health education and promotion, including the Office of Education, the Consumer Product Safety Commission, the Department of Agriculture, the Environmental Protection Agency, the National Institutes of Health, the Department of Transportation, and the Department of Defense; and

(3) identify Federal programs and actions which are not in the interest of public health and determine methods for reviewing and commenting on such programs and actions.

Section 104 establishes an Interdepartmental Committee on Health Education and Promotion to promote and maintain the effectiveness of Federal health education programs. The Secretary will chair the committee and the remainder of the committee shall be appointed by the President from among heads of Federal departments engaged in health education activities.

Section 105 (a) establishes the Health Education and Promotion Advisory Council. The Council shall consist of 19 members appointed by the Secretary and the Secretary shall appoint from time to time the chairman of the council. The Section establishes the categories of representation on the council, the tenure of members, procedures for appointing members where a council member vacates his appointment prematurely, member pay entitlements for serving and for certain expenses, and matters related to the calling of meetings.

Section 105 (b) provides that the council will advise the Secretary and make recommendations to him on matters of general policy with respect to the functions of the Center. The council shall make an annual report to the Secretary and to Congress relating to the performance of its functions and any recommendations it may have with respect thereto.

Section 105 (c) authorizes the council to engage any technical assistance that may be required to carry out its functions and requires the Secretary to make available to the council the necessary clerical, secretarial and administrative support, and to provide pertinent data available to the Department of Health, Education, and Welfare which the council might need to carry out its functions.

Section 106 prescribes the contents of the annual reports that must be submitted by the Secretary to the President and to Congress. The Secretary, acting through the Center, shall submit such reports not later than December 1 of each year.

Section 107 authorizes appropriation of $35,000,000 for fiscal year 1976, and $40,000,000 for fiscal year 1977, and $45,000,000 for 1978.

Title II. Institution for Health Education and Promotion

Section 201 states that the Congress finds and declares that:

(1)   it is in the public interest to inform the public about health and about ways to best protect and improve personal health;

(2)   the public must develop the ability to examine and weigh consequences of personal decisions respecting health;

(3)   the public must be motivated to desire changes supportive of more healthful life-styles;

(4)   impediments that inhibit the voluntary adoption and maintenance of more healthful practices by the public must be identified and mitigated or removed;

(5)   to achieve these goals it is necessary for the Federal Government to complement, assist, and support a national policy that will advance the national health, reduce preventable illness, disability, and death, moderate self-imposed risks, and promote progress and scholarship in consumer health education and preventive medicine; and

(6)   a private corporation should be created to facilitate the development of a health education and promotion strategy for the nation.

Section 202 establishes a not-for-profit-corporation to be known as the Institution for Health Education and Promotion. The institution shall not be an agency or establishment of the United States Government.

Section 203 (a) provides that the corporation shall have a twenty-five member board of directors appointed by the President with the advice and consent of the Senate.

Section 203 (b) provides that the board shall have broad representation of the various regions of the country and of the various skills and experiences appropriate to the functions and responsibilities of the Institution.

Section 203 (c) provides that the members of the initial board shall also serve as its incorporators and are charged with taking whatever actions are necessary to establish the Institution under the District of Columbia Nonprofit Corporation Act.

Section 203 (d) establishes the terms of office for board members, procedures to be followed when a member leaves the board prematurely, and provisions for staggering the terms of office of the original board members. The Section provides that no board member shall serve for more than two consecutive terms.

Section 203 (e) provides that any vacancy in the Board shall not effect its power, and the vacancy shall be filled in the same manner in which the original appointments were made.

Section 203 (f) establishes procedures for appointment of officers by the Board of Directors.

Section 203 (g) provides that the members of the Board of Directors shall not be deemed Federal employees by reason of the membership on the Board, and provides for payment for their time and travel expenses related to Board meetings and other activities of the Board.

Section 204 (a) provides that the Institution shall have a President and other officers that may be appointed by the Board. The Board will determine the terms and rates of compensation of those appointed. No officer, other than the Chairman, and vice chairman, may receive any salary or other compensation from any source other than the Institution during their employment. The officers shall serve at the pleasure of the Board.

Section 204 (b) provides that no political test or qualification shall be used in selecting, appointing, promoting, or taking other personnel actions with respect to officers, agents, and employees of the Institution.

Section 205 (a) provides that the Institution strategy for the nation, the Institution of stock or to declare or pay dividends.

Section 205 (b) provides that no part of the income or assets of the Institution shall insure to the benefit of any director, officer, employee, or any other individual except as salary or other reasonable compensation for services.

Section 205 (c) provides that the Institution may not contribute to or otherwise support any political party or candidate for elective office.

Section 206 states that to facilitate the development of a health education and promotion strategy for the nation, the Institution shall carry out the following functions:

(1) Establish communications with, provide a forum for the involvement of, and seek the advice and support of, organizations, agencies, and groups involved in health care, education, labor and business, social and civic organizations, consumer organizations, and communications. The Institution shall review and analyze the need, and resources available, for health education and promotion and the effect of alternative health education methods and procedures on health status to determine which methods and procedures offer the best opportunities for improving the nation's health.

(2) Coordinate and stimulate a variety of projects involving other organizations, agencies, and groups to develop such strategy designs or design components as are required to increase the appropriateness, acceptability, and effectiveness of health education efforts nationwide.

(3) Assist in stimulating, developing, implementing, and assessing a total communications program utilizing a full range of media available to

reach diversified groups in order to increase national understanding and support for the value of health education and the role each citizen and every organization, institution, and agency can and should play to improve individual, community, and, ultimately, the national health through educational means.

(4)   Assist in accelerating the incorporation of improved technology into health education practice by establishing a system of technical assistance and training and by making available the expertise of other cooperating organizations, as well as its own staff, in response to the needs of national, State, and local groups for assistance in improving the planning, implementation, and evaluation of their health education programs.

(5)   Encourage the development and utilization of valid and acceptable research and evaluation methods for a wide variety of health education programs and technologies. It shall develop coalitions and consortium arrangements with other organizations and agencies for cooperative efforts in model design and testing and for joint sponsorship and exchange of information on comparable research and evaluation projects.

Section 207 provides that the Board shall appoint an advisory panel of 200 individuals with appropriate competencies and abilities. Its principal function will be to advise the Board. The panel shall also serve as a resource of appointments to special committees, task forces, and conferences. The advisory panel shall receive all Institution reports.

Section 208 requires the Institution to submit an annual report to the President for transmittal to Congress. The report shall include a detailed account of the activities of the Institution, its operations, financial condition and accomplishments. Additionally, it may include such recommendations as the Institution deems appropriate.

Section 209 authorizes appropriations for expenses of the Institution of $1,000,000 in fiscal year 1976, $3,000,000 in fiscal year 1977, and $5,000,000 in fiscal year 1978.

Section 210 (a) provides that the accounts of the Institution shall be audited annually in accordance with generally accepted auditing standards by independent public accountants certified or licensed by a regulatory authority of a State or other political subdivision of the United States. The Section also provides that the audit will occur at the place where the accounts of the Institution are normally kept.

Section 210 (b) provides that the auditor's report shall be included in the annual report required by Section 208. This Section also describes the contents of the auditors' report as it would be displayed in the Institution's annual report required under Section 208.

Appendix U
NIH-Fogarty International Center—ACPM
Expert Panel on Consumer Health Education

Anne R. Somers, Chairman
Professor of Community Medicine
and Family Medicine
College of Medicine & Dentistry of
New Jersey—Rutgers Medical School
Piscataway, New Jersey 08854

Frederic Bass, M.D., D.Sc.
Vancouver Health Department
1060 West 8th Avenue
Vancouver, B.C.
Canada, V6H 1C4

John Davidson, M.D.
Professor of Medicine
Director, Diabetes Unit
Emory School of Medicine
Atlanta, Georgia 30303

Joy Dryfoos
Director of Planning
The Alan Guttmacher Institute
515 Madison Avenue
New York, New York 10022

Thomas D. Dublin, M.D.
6907 Bradley Boulevard
Bethesda, Maryland 20034

Lawrence W. Green, Dr. P.H.
Head, Division of Health
   Education
School of Hygiene and Public
   Health
Johns Hopkins University
Baltimore, Maryland 21205

Godfrey M. Hochbaum, Ph.D.
Professor of Health Education
School of Public Health
University of North Carolina
Chapel Hill, North Carolina 27514

Barbara Lee, R.N.
Program Director
Kellogg Foundation
400 North Avenue
Battle Creek, Michigan 49016

223

Nathan Maccoby, Ph.D.
Chairman, Institute of
    Communication Research
Co-Director, Stanford Heart
    Disease Prevention Program
Stanford University Medical
    Center
Stanford, California 94305

Carter L. Marshall, M.D.
Associate Dean
Mt. Sinai School of Medicine
The City University of New York
Fifth Avenue and 100th Street
New York, New York 10029

Richard N. Podell, M.D., M.P.H.
Associate Director of Family
    Practice Training
Overlook Hospital
193 Morris Avenue
Summit, New Jersey 07901

Henry Simmons, M.D.
Senior Vice-President
J. Walter Thompson Company
420 Lexington Avenue
New York, New York 10017

Scott K. Simonds, Dr. P.H.
Professor of Health Education
School of Public Health
University of Michigan
Ann Arbor, Michigan 48104

Arthur J. Viseltear, Ph.D.
Associate Professor
Department of Epidemiology and
    Public Health
Yale University
School of Medicine
New Haven, Connecticut 06510

EX OFFICIO

Shirley Bagley
Health Scientist Administrator
National Institute of Aging
Landow Building, Room A810
Bethesda, Maryland 20014

Donald Carmody
Director, Division of Health
    Protection
Office of Policy Development and
    Planning
Office of the Assistant Secretary
    for Health
Parklawn Building, Room 17A31
5600 Fishers Lane
Rockville, Maryland 20852

Lois K. Cohen, Ph.D.
Special Assistant to the Director
Division of Dentistry
Bureau of Health Manpower—
    HRA
Federal Building, Room 3C–10
7550 Wisconsin Avenue
Bethesda, Maryland 20014

Delbert Dayton, M.D.
Pediatrician
Growth and Development Branch
NICHD
Landow Building, Room C716
Bethesda, Maryland 20014

Edward Friedlander
Special Assistant
Office of the Commissioner
Food and Drug Administration
Parklawn Building
5600 Fishers Lane
Rockville, Maryland 20852

Maurice Glatzer
Bureau of Health Education
Center for Disease Control
Atlanta, Georgia 30333

Alice Horowitz
National Institute of Dental
   Research
Westwood Building
Bethesda, Maryland 20014

Ms. Susan M. Horowitz
Program Analyst
Division of Medicine
Bureau of Health Manpower
Building 31, Room 3C33
Bethesda, Maryland 20014

Dr. Keatha K. Krueger
Director, Diabetes Program
NIAMDD

Westwood Building, Room 626A
Bethesda, Maryland 20014

Carl A. Larson, Ed.D.
Program Director for Special
   Educational Projects
Division of Cancer Control and
   Rehabilitation
National Cancer Institute
Blair Building, Room 732B
Bethesda, Maryland 20014

Arthur J. McDowell
Director, Division of Health
   Examination Studies
National Center for Health
   Statistics
Parklawn Building, Room 8A54
5600 Fishers Lane
Rockville, Maryland 20852

Dr. Jim L. Shields
Assistant Director for Health
   Information Programs
Office of Prevention, Control and
   Education
NHLI
Building 31, Room 5A10
Bethesda, Maryland 20014

Appendix V
Prevention
Excerpted from *Forward Plan for Health, FY 1977–81*
U.S. Department of Health, Education, and Welfare, PHS
June 1975

INTRODUCTION

Public Health and preventive medicine have made many contributions to the conquest of disease. The success of efforts to rid this country of smallpox and to control the childhood diseases attest to the efficacy of immunization. Similarly, the benefits of requiring the pasteurization of milk and of modern plumbing and waste treatment plants in the control of diseases such as typhoid are well-known.

Comparisons of the leading causes of death in 1900 and today dramatize the major changes that have occurred in the nature of the problems we now face and, therefore, in the way we must deal with them. The earlier killers, pneumonia, influenza, and tuberculosis, have been supplanted by diseases of the heart and malignant neoplasms. Tuberculosis ranks 21 on the list of causes of death. Can public health in the last quarter of this century mount as successful an attack on the chronic diseases as it has on the communicable?

Many of today's health problems are caused by a variety of factors not susceptible to medical solutions or to direct intervention by the health practitioner: we have as yet no vaccine to prevent cancer or to cure alcoholism. This poses a dilemma for health professionals in defining a proper role for themselves in the prevention of disease and a practical problem for those concerned with setting the boundaries of health planning. For planning purposes, for example, it is not realistic to view smoking primarily as a medical problem. It is a major social, economic, cultural, and psychological phenomenon that has profound health implications.

Similarly, the annual carnage on our highways generates costly demands on the health care system but the behavior of the individual behind the wheel

227

of a speeding car and the condition of the car and highway are determined by social, cultural, and economic factors that have little direct involvement with the health professions.

In the area of the environment we are seeing increasingly persuasive evidence linking a range of human diseases to our industrial society. Failure to deal with this contamination of our environment could result in serious health consequences whose full effects may not be known for decades to come. Clearly this requires attention and action on a scale going far beyond the borders of medicine.

While scientists do not yet agree on the specific casual relationships, evidence is mounting that the kinds and amount of food and liquor we consume and the style of living common in our generally affluent, sedentary society are major factors associated with cancer, cardiovascular disease, and other chronic illnesses.

Given these facts, the question arises: who should be primarily responsible for viewing such health-related problems in their entirety and for devising comprehensive proposals for action? While we cannot answer that question completely, we do assert that the Public Health Service has a duty to assess such problems in their broadest terms and to propose solutions whether or not this Department, the Federal Government, States and localities, or the private sector is the most appropriate locus for dealing with them.

Approaches to Prevention

Prevention is often described as consisting of three stages: primary, secondary, and tertiary prevention. Primary prevention includes actions or interventions designed to prevent etiologic agents from causing disease or injury in man. Secondary prevention is concerned with the early detection and treatment of disease in order to cure or control its course. Tertiary prevention includes those activities directed at ameliorating the seriousness of disease by reducing disability and dependence resulting from it.

For planning purposes, we believe it is more productive to focus our attention on the underlying conditions or antecedent causes of preventable diseases than to concentrate on the diseases themselves. For example, by reviewing the dimensions of the problems of cigarette smoking, alcoholism, and toxic chemicals in the workplace (rather than lung cancer or cardiovascular diseases) we can fashion program goals and initiatives more carefully aimed at basic causes. This approach also provides a broader framework within which to analyze problems and to consider a range of medical, legislative, regulatory and economic alternatives that may not fit within the usual medical model. (We are indebted to the Canadian Minister of National Health and Welfare for this and other insights discussed in the publication,

A New Perspective on the Health of Canadians: A Working Document. Ottawa, Government of Canada, 1974.)

While we propose that a higher priority be given to the development of primary prevention programs directed at the underlying causes of disease, we recognize that in some instances our capacity to affect these problems is limited or unknown. Many of them involve fundamental changes in the behavior of people and in the traditional practices of social and economic institutions. It would be unrealistic to expect significant improvements within a short time. Efforts will therefore continue to be directed toward improving the scope and utility of prevention programs for the early detection and treatment of disease and for the reduction of disability and dependence. This must be accompanied by an assessment of the efficacy and costs of all preventive approaches. During the past year under the sponsorship of the Fogarty Center for International Health at NIH, Task Forces reviewed the State of the Art of Prevention. Some of their preliminary conclusions are summarized in Appendix II.

We can only begin to suggest in this document the actions needed and the initial role which the Federal Government can play. A basic assumption underlying our approach is that despite major gaps in our knowledge, enough is known about the links between these diseases and their antecedent conditions to justify a special emphasis on primary preventive action now.

Central to our perception of these problems is the knowledge that they are no longer inexplicable events which we cannot avert. An overwhelming portion of them are caused by man and his institutions and can, theoretically, be prevented or controlled by man. Perhaps more important at this time than agreement on specific proposals is the explicit commitment of the Public Health Service and the Secretary of HEW to the goals of primary prevention and the determination to apply the energies and resources of this Department to help find practical ways of achieving those goals.

It is worth noting that some of the important prevention objectives depend in part on individuals deciding to change their style of living—for example, to stop smoking, exercise more, or reduce their liquor consumption. The question arises, then, about government's role in this process. While there can probably be no entirely satisfactory philosophic answer to that question, it is clear that the government's function is to enable people to make sound decisions about their health, to equip them with the information and skills and other resources to translate these decisions into action, and to aid in the removal of legal, economic, physical, or other barriers that might prevent them from acting accordingly. Therefore, where this Theme suggests options for action which depend on changes in people's behavior, it should be understood that as far as government actions are concerned the proposals are intended solely to provide opportunities and incentives for people to assume full responsibility for their own health. Even so, it is clearly appropriate to provide for public discussion of such options.

I. PREVENTABLE HEALTH PROBLEMS AND OPTIONS FOR ACTION

The ultimate goal of a prevention strategy is to enable each person to live long and free from disability by reducing the occurrence of disease or injury.

The following sections summarize some of what is known about the antecedent causes of or factors associated with the principal diseases afflicting the United States today. Each of them is thought to be responsible for or contribute to a range of maladies, and their prevention or control could significantly improve the health status of large segments of the population.

After each summary is a listing of options for action to attack these problems. These are not limited to actions that could be undertaken by the Public Health Service, nor does listing them imply that PHS advocates any particular option. Rather, a wide range of alternatives is considered, irrespective of what agency, level of government or group in the private sector is best fitted to carry them out.

The feasibility, efficacy, cost benefits, and consequences of the proposals should be fully assessed by professional and community groups. Decisions to undertake some of them probably require action through political or budgetary processes. In other instances, changes in institutional program emphases would be sufficient.

A. Smoking

1. The Problem

According to the Federal Trade Commission, the per capita consumption of cigarettes for the eighteen and older population for 1974 was 4,270, the highest since 1963, the year before the Surgeon General's Report. Since 1964 there has been a decline in smoking in the 25 and older population, particularly among men, but teenage smoking levels, especially for women, have increased.

There is strong evidence that smoking-related diseases include cancer of the lung, larynx, lip, oral cavity, esophagus, bladder and other urinary organs; chronic bronchitis and emphysema; arteriosclerotic heart disease, including coronary artery disease; and specified non-coronary cardiovascular diseases. The President's Science Advisory Committee in its 1973 report, *Chemicals and Health*, estimated that in 1967, 16 percent of the total mortality could be linked to cigarette smoking. The 1967 Public Health Service Report, *Cigarette Smoking and Health*, noted that in general, the more cigarettes a person smoked, the more days of illness he was likely to have.

2. Options

Legislation/Enforcement/Regulation

- Make the warning label on cigarette packages more explicit about the disease risks, and the regulations more specific concerning the size and prominence of the warning statement in advertising.
- Consider restricting the sale of cigarettes with high tar and nicotine content.
- Phase out tobacco price supports and eliminate cigarettes from the "Food for Peace" program.
- Ban cigarette advertisements or exclude such advertising as a deductible business expense for tax purposes.
- Encourage the Federal Trade Communications Commission to require that prime time be available for anti-smoking spots on television and radio.

Behavior Change

- Intensify anti-smoking campaigns, particularly for such target groups as youth, women, adults with high risk of disease, and workers in industries in which the combination of industrial exposure and smoking creates special risks.
- Continue to emphasize the dangers of smoking in school health education programs, especially those aimed at elementary school students.
- Encourage and financially support programs to aid those who are trying to give up smoking.

Incentive

- Raise the Federal excise tax on cigarettes, either uniformly on all cigarettes or differentially based on the level of tar and nicotine content.

Research

- Expand efforts to develop a cigarette substitute or a safe cigarette.
- Conduct further research on techniques to assist people to stop smoking.

B. Alcohol

1. The Problem

The consumption of alcohol permeates our society. More than 100 million Americans are drinkers, and nine million of them are classified as alcoholics or alcohol abusers. Alcohol plays a role in half of the Nation's highway fatalities, half of all homicides, and one third of the suicides. The cost to society is more than $15 billion in lost work time, health and welfare services, and property damage.

While moderate drinking apparently does little or no harm, its abuse takes a significant toll. Cirrhosis of the liver is a major cause of illness and death in alcoholics, and excessive use of alcohol, especially when combined with smoking, increases the risk of developing certain cancers. Other serious problems include: malnutrition; lowered resistance to infectious disease; gastrointestinal irritations; muscle diseases and tremors; and damage to the brain or peripheral nervous system. Abuse during pregnancy has serious health effects on the offspring, and the significance of heredity in alcoholism is as yet unresolved.

2. Options

Legislation/Regulation/Enforcement
- Develop consistent State and local alcohol control laws oriented towards prevention of abuse.
- Increase communication between control agencies and those agencies involved with alcohol-related problems.
- Reduce the alcohol content of certain beverages.
- Restrict advertisements for alcoholic beverages or exclude such advertising as a deductible business expense for tax purposes.

Incentive
- Adjust the tax rate according to the amount of absolute alcohol in the beverage.

Behavior Change
- Develop cooperative educational programs on the limits of responsible drinking, identification of problem drinkers, and availability of community resources.
- Target special educational efforts at school children, health professionals, and children of alcoholic parents.

Health Maintenance
- Give special support to programs effective in early detection, and to treatment services designed to meet the needs of those in earlier stages of alcohol-related problems.

Research
Research needs include:
- Evaluation of the effect of State and local regulations in fostering alcohol abuse.
- Greater understanding of the relationship of alcohol use to: various disease states; pregnancy and fetal health; and genetic and environmental influences on the addictive process.
- The development of more effective health education methodologies suitable to the field of alcohol abuse.

C. Inadequate or Excessive Food Consumption

1. The Problem

Nutritional problems range from malnutrition and "dietary subnutrition," to obesity due to overeating, to the quality and safety of the food supply.

Malnutrition can be a cause of fetal immaturity and prematurity, and some studies have demonstrated an association between poor nutrition in pregnant women and retardation in the development of the fetus, particularly of the brain. Among young children, malnutrition is often associated with learning disability.

Malnutrition is more often found in poverty areas and among the aged who are often unable to purchase, prepare, or ingest adequate meals—resulting in conditions such as subnutrition, obesity, atherosclerosis, vitamin deficiencies, anemia, and diabetes.

Obesity, which may affect as much as 30 percent of Americans, is directly related to increased risk of mortality and with heightened susceptibility to diabetes, hypertension, arthritis, pulmonary dysfunction, angina, gall bladder disease, and increased complications and mortality from surgery.

Coronary heart disease appears to be associated with modern dietary habits, especially increased intake of saturated fats and cholesterol. There is extensive evidence of the crucial role of dietary fats in the initiation and progression of atherosclerotic vascular disease. Sizable reductions in incidence of new coronary heart disease events have been achieved with fat-modified diets. Diet is also a major factor in the prevention and reduction of hypertension.

Although the relationship between dietary intake and cancer is not fully understood, an association has been established, especially with cancers of the digestive organs. There is also a correlation between the prevalence of diabetes and the general level and standard of dietary intake, with an impressive association between obesity and diabetes. Sugar ingestion, by promoting dental decay, is a major dietary factor affecting dental health.

Health problems also result from hazardous substances in food. Potentials for hazard exist with additives, fortifiers, artificial colors and flavors, as well as with inadvertent contaminants, infectious agents, naturally occurring toxins, and other dangerous materials.

2. Options

Legislation/Regulation/Enforcement
- Expand efforts to monitor and analyze the nutrient composition of foods and of potentially harmful substances in food.

- Develop strong regulations to control the advertisement of food products, especially those of high sugar content or little nutritive value. Children's TV would be a special focus of such efforts. Also establish strict regulations concerning food labelling, and require full disclosure of contents.
- Explore the merits, feasibility, and need for mandatory open dating of certain perishable foods.

Incentives
- Base life and health insurance premiums on weight standards, with higher premiums for those significantly in excess of their ideal weight.

Behavior Change
- Develop nutrition education programs to help the public at large and special high risk populations to select suitable foods.

Health Maintenance
- Make nutrition concerns a mandatory component of all DHEW health activities. Include nutrition and health concerns in the policy development processes of all DHEW agencies and of other Federal agencies.
- Strengthen monitoring activities to establish nutritional status, eating habits, and relationship of consumption to various health states.

Research
- Focus research on explicating the role of nutrition in the prevention of disease, determination of nutrient requirements, behavioral aspects of nutrition, methods of appraising nutritional status, and nutrition education methodologies.

D. Motor Vehicle Accidents

1. The Problem

In 1973 motor vehicle accidents accounted for 55,800 deaths and an estimated 2,000,000 disabling injuries. They are the leading cause of death of those between the ages of 5 and 35.

Improper driving (including speeding) and alcohol and drug abuse were major contributing factors. Studies by the National Safety Council have concluded that reduced speeds, particularly the 55 m.p.h. limit, saved approximately 5,600 lives in 1973–1974. The Council estimates that if drunken driving were controlled one half of the fatalities could be eliminated.

Seat belts, if everyone wore them, could save an estimated 14,000 lives or 25 percent of the annual motor vehicle fatalities.

2. Options

Legislation/Enforcement/Regulation
- Continue and strictly enforce the 55-mile per hour speed limit.

- Increase legal penalties for driving under the influence of alcohol. Require those who are convicted of drunken driving, and any driver with a certain number of violations, to reapply for a license every 6 months and enroll in a safe driving program. Expand treatment programs as alternatives to jail or fines for those convicted of drunken driving.
- Require all drivers and passengers to wear safety belts at all times.

Modifying the Environment
- Improve road conditions. Careful engineering of roadways, well marked areas of danger, and good lighting are essential to the safe operation of cars.
- Continue efforts to design a safer automobile, with particular emphasis on such modifications as the air bag.

Behavior Change
- Expand and improve safe driving programs in the schools and media campaigns, giving special attention to the drunk driver and the teenage driver.
- Expand education and behavior improvement services for drinking drivers.

Incentives
- Reduce insurance premiums for those with good driving records.
- Give financial incentives to companies that develop safety devices.

E. Environmental Pollution

1. The Problem

Urbanization, industrialization, rising population, increased agricultural output, technological advancement and need for new and more energy sources are creating an exponential increase in the chemical pollution of our food, air, and water. While the acute toxicological properties of these pollutants are often well-known, the long-term health effects and chronic toxicity of many of these chemicals are as yet not established.

Epidemiologic studies have repeatedly shown a greater prevalence of chronic bronchitis, emphysema, respiratory infections and lung cancer in residents of heavily polluted urban areas than is found in rural residents.

Modern water treatment plants and the extensive use of chlorine have reduced the incidence of waterborne infections. However, treatment plants must contend with an increasing variety and quantity of compounds associated with industrial, agricultural, and domestic wastes. The effects of these compounds—only a small number of which have been identified and studied—may not become evident for decades.

Pesticides and other new synthetic organic compounds are especially dangerous because of their acute and chronic toxicity, their ability to disrupt the food chain, and to enter into it through food and water processing.

2. Options

Legislation/Regulation/Enforcement
- Formally clarify the Departmental policy on the health aspects of the environment so that a more systematic, coordinated research and regulatory effort can be undertaken between PHS and such agencies as EPA.
- Encourage legislation to form a nationwide environmental monitoring network.
- Encourage the passage of legislation to control toxic substances and explore the practicality of establishing a premarketing safety clearance or "early warning" system for new substances and their degradation products.
- Establish a joint programming effort between EPA and PHS to determine total exposure and body burden levels of toxic substances and effective programs to control such exposures in food, water, and air.

Incentives
- Encourage private organizations and industry to develop technology to identify and reduce harmful pollutants.
- Give special funding priority to epidemiological studies to detect pollutant-related effects in urban industrial areas.

Behavior Change
- Expand educational activities in industry, universities, and school systems on the health effects of environmental pollutants.
- Promote programs designed to alert government, industry, and the general public to the hazards of environmental pollution and of the ways to prevent it.

Research
Continue efforts to:
- Determine the additive and synergistic effects of pollutants.
- Expand activity to identify the prevalence of toxic substances in food, water, and air and determine the total exposure and body burden of the public to these substances.
- Study the carcinogenic, mutagenic, and teratogenic effects of long-term, low-level doses of chemical pollutants.
- Develop more rapid, predictable tests for long-term effects of pollutants on health.
- Ensure that the design and operation of new sources of energy do not impose excessive health burdens.
- Establish priorities for research based on prevalence and persistence of environmental substances and their potential toxicity.

F. Physical Inactivity

1. The Problem

According to the President's Council on Physical Fitness and Sports, the American sedentary way of life constitutes a serious national health problem, particularly for the 45 percent of all American adults who never exercise. Habitual physical inactivity is thought to contribute to hypertension, chronic fatigue and resulting physical inefficiency, premature aging, the poor musculature and lack of flexibility that are the major causes of lower back pain and injury, mental tension, coronary heart disease, and obesity.

By contrast, studies have reported that regular exercise can lower serum triglycerides, reduce the clinical manifestations of heart disease, improve the efficiency of the heart and circulation, and reduce blood pressure levels in individuals with hypertension.

In 1971, the National Heart and Lung Institute Task Force on Arteriosclerosis stated that preliminary incomplete evidence indicated that regular exercise may decrease either the rate of development of arteriosclerosis or its consequences.

2. Options

Health Maintenance
- Encourage physicians to stress the importance of physical activity to patients and, when necessary, prescribe a regimen of activities. According to one poll, four of every five Americans say they have never been advised to exercise by a physician.

Modifying the Environment
- Provide an environment that makes it easier to engage in safe physical activity. Communities, for example, could build paths for jogging, bicycling, and walking. Pools could be made more accessible, and places of work could be encouraged to provide facilities and time for employees to participate in individual or group fitness activities.

Behavior Change
- Expand information campaigns to warn the public of the health hazards of sedentary living.
- In physical education programs for elementary, junior, and senior high school students, stress the health benefits of and ways to continue physical fitness activities as adults.

Research
- Encourage competent research to obtain more authoritative information on the role of physical activity in maintaining health and preventing disease, particularly cardiovascular disease.

Incentives
  ● Strengthen and expand programs recognizing achievement in physical fitness.

G. Diseases and Injuries of the Workplace

1. The Problem

Occupational injuries and diseases pose a major, continuing threat to the health of American workers. About 14,000 workers are killed each year in work accidents and more than 2.2 million more are either permanently or temporarily disabled as a result of work accidents and occupational disease. It has been estimated that almost 500,000 workers develop occupational diseases each year and that as high as 100,000 deaths might be associated with occupational disease. A recent preliminary study suggests that diseases suffered by three of every ten factory or farm workers are caused by work conditions, and that 90 percent of the work-related health conditions are not reported. The total loss to the GNP each year is in excess of $9 billion.

In addition to overt diseases due to lead and mercury poisoning and the insidious effects of noise and dust, exposure to some occupational hazards can cause or contribute to the development of cancer and hasten the onset of certain degenerative diseases. It has also been shown that families of workers exposed to certain disease-producing substances have higher incidence rates of those diseases than the general population. Approximately fifteen thousand chemicals are commonly used in industry and about 3,000 new ones are developed each year. The potential health hazards of these chemicals are unknown.

2. Options

Legislation/Regulation/Enforcement
  ● Enact National health insurance legislation which encourages employers to establish effective occupational health and safety programs.

Incentives
  ● Encourage insurance companies to make greater use of experience ratings to induce employers to provide healthier working environments.
  ● Allow employers to receive tax benefits for engineering changes that assure a healthier work environment for the employees and reduce the need for him to use protective equipment or clothing.

Behavior Change
  ● Expand opportunities for the training of workers and their union representatives in occupational health and safety.
  ● Inform employees (including non-union employees) of their rights under the OSHA Act, including requests for health hazard surveys.

- Promote balanced information campaigns to alert the public and the worker to the hazards of the workplace and what can be done to reduce them.

Health Maintenance

- Encourage small industries to collaborate in the provision of comprehensive health and safety programs.
- Improve epidemiological surveys and reporting systems to determine occupational disease and injury etiology.
- Use NIOSH research findings to give the public early warning of environmental exposure hazards.

Research

Focus research efforts on:

- Employee behavior patterns in the work setting.
- Work-related cancer and chronic illness.
- The effects of exposure to family members to materials introduced into the household by industrial workers.
- The synergistic effects of chemical substances in the work setting.

H. Infectious Diseases

1. The Problem

Among the leading microbial causes of death and morbidity, six major categories account for a large percentage of infectious disease incidence. They are: venereal diseases (gonorrhea, with an estimated annual incidence of 2.5 million cases, ranks first among the reportable diseases); viral infections of the respiratory tract (these probably account for 60 percent of all non-fatal illnesses and are responsible for 65,000 to 100,000 deaths per year); hepatitis (it is estimated that 500,000 cases of hepatitis A and 162,000 cases of hepatitis B occurred in 1970); nosocomial infections (which strike approximately 5 percent of all patients admitted to our hospitals); infectious diseases preventable by immunization; and enteric diseases (salmonellosis, shigellosis, botulism, etc.). The prevention and control of infectious diseases has long been a goal of National and local disease control efforts.

2. Options

Elimination of Vaccine-Preventable Diseases

- Continue community immunization programs for childhood diseases.
- Maintain adequate outbreak control programs throughout the country.
- Continue to emphasize the information-education-motivation component of immunization delivery systems.
- Explore the merits of Federal legislation compensating the rare victim of vaccine-produced illness.

- Establish an in-place immunization delivery system to take advantage of new vaccines as they are developed—e.g., promising work in hepatitis B and live virus influenza vaccines.
- Reassess the scientific merits of influenza vaccination programs for high risk groups, including the elderly.

Venereal Diseases

- Develop disease interruption activities—primarily casefinding and contact follow-up, screening by culture of persons with asymptomatic gonorrhea, and information and education activities.
- Initiate or expand outreach efforts by States and cities to identify persons in need of treatment.
- Increase public awareness and communication of pertinent VD facts to people at risk, especially youth.

Diagnostic Capability of Clinical Laboratories

- Achieve uniformity of quality control standards, including proficiency testing, for all clinical laboratories under the authority of DHEW.
- Upgrade the capacity of State laboratories to carry out active quality control and inspection programs of laboratories within the State.
- Provide specialized technical consultation, short-term training, and information on latest laboratory technologies and procedures.

I. Product Safety

1. The Problem

a. Food-Related Illness and Deaths

Between two and 20 million cases of food poisoning occur each year in this country. Microbiological contamination of food affects more people than any other food-related problem. Prime factors contributing to food poisoning are the increase in home canning of foods, poor food handling practices within the home, the growing practice of eating foods prepared outside the home, and the increasing use of convenience foods. Another factor is the lack of proper equipment and inadequate production and storage practices in many food processing establishments.

Another form of food contamination is caused by mycotoxins, which are produced by molds growing on food under certain temperature and moisture conditions. These molds form because of inadequate growing, storage, or processing practices.

Environmental pollution is another source of food contamination. The short-term toxicological significance of some heavy metals and industrial chemicals is already known, but information on the long-term effects of low levels of environmental contaminants in a wide range of foods is inadequate.

Deleterious chemicals may become constituents of food in a number of ways, including migration from food packaging or from the surface coatings of food handling equipment. The safety of substances, such as polyvinyl chloride (a plasticizer), which may migrate to foods from packaging, must also be reviewed to assure safety.

b. Medical Device and Diagnostic Product Injuries and Deaths

The application of any therapeutic or diagnostic device involves some inherent potential risk to the patient because of a manufacturing defect, operator error, or an adverse environmental condition. In the last year, FDA has encountered serious product defects in such life-sustaining devices as cardiac pacemakers, heart valves, arterial shunts, oxygen delivery systems, defibrillators, catheters, and hemodialysis units. Precise data on the number of injuries caused by faulty medical devices are not available at present.

c. Drugs and Biologics

It is estimated that over 225 million prescriptions were written in 1974. Many of these drugs have been found to be sub-potent, or super-potent, contaminated with other drugs, and compounded with the wrong ingredients. Parenteral drugs contaminated with pathogenic microorganisms have caused serious injuries and deaths.

Drugs have become an intrinsic part of medical treatment and disease management. The average practicing physician has been reported to prescribe some pharmacological agent for 75 percent of his patients. While the benefits of relevant drug therapy have been amply publicized, the occurrence of unwanted effects associated with their use have only recently been the subject of quantitative investigation.

Studies have shown that 5 percent of patients admitted to a general medical service in a major university hospital did so because of a drug reaction, and that once hospitalized, there was a 10 to 30 percent chance of acquiring another adverse drug reaction. Additional data suggest that this figure is matched, or possibly exceeded, in pediatric populations.

In 1974, an HEW study group agreed that "the widespread availability of antibiotics has clearly played a role in the increasing incidence of gram-negative rod bacteremia." The group noted, however, that other factors such as the large proportion of elderly in hospitals, greater use of immunosuppressive agents, and poor infection control procedures also contribute to increased gram-negative rod bacteremia infections.

d. Radiation Injury and Death

The principal source of man-made ionizing radiation, accounting for more than 90 percent of the exposure of the population, is the X-ray machine used for diagnostic and therapeutic purposes.

Biological effects from radiation exposure include death, genetic mutations, cancer, birth defects, cataracts, and other non-specific life shortening effects. In November 1972, the National Academy of Sciences/National Research Council issued a report pointing out that much of today's medical X-ray exposure is unnecessary and can be significantly reduced through simple improvements in the techniques of X-ray users.

Largely due to ignorance of available radiation protection techniques, radiation exposure of patients in many hospitals and offices is needlessly high. For example, survey data show that radiation doses to the male reproductive organs resulting from X-ray examinations of the lower back is 2,000 times higher in some facilities than in others depending upon the protective techniques employed.

The National Academy of Sciences (NAS) has quantified ionizing radiation exposure and estimated its associated biological effects. Application of the NAS estimates of avoidable medical radiation exposure indicates that a possible 1,800 cancer deaths occur annually because of unnecessary exposure and that ill-health due to X-ray induced genetic damage accounts for approximately 2 percent of direct health care costs.

e. Viral Hepatitis

The transmission of viral hepatitis B from blood donors to blood recipients is estimated to occur in 20,000 to 30,000 transfused patients with a fatal outcome in 800 to 2,000 patients annually. Testing methods available to blood banks over the past 2 years have only been able to identify about 25 percent of hepatitis contaminated blood. In addition, some blood banks and plasmapheresis centers fail to control adequately their various blood processing operations.

2. Options

Food

- Significantly increase the surveillance of those food commodities that have a high hazard potential.
- Develop rapid screening drug residue detection methods for the largest volume drugs used in food-producing animals.

Medical Devices and Diagnostic Products

- Establish standards for the highest priority medical devices and diagnostic products.
- Inspect all medical device firms every two years with special investigations as needed.
- Initiate, when the legislation passes, the scientific review process for new medical devices.
- Conduct the necessary bioeffect and methods development research that will be needed to support FDA's regulatory process in the medical device area.

Drugs and Biologics

- Conduct comprehensive GMP inspections of all drug plants every two years.

- Conduct an intensive surveillance of all potentially high risk drugs.
- Implement fully the National Blood Program established by the President in 1972–1973.
- Develop a National Prescription Drug Compendium.
- Update and revise FDA's procedural and product regulations, many of which will have to be revised as a result of the findings of the biologic safety and efficacy review panels.
- Revise all testing protocols and increase product testing of biologics prior to release.
- Implement the recommendations of the NAS Conference on Adverse Drug Reaction Reporting System.

Radiation
- Increase the surveillance of new diagnostic X-ray installations by FDA and State inspectors.
- Support the development of new X-ray technologies that can eventually reduce X-ray exposure by a factor of 10 or more.
- Develop X-ray ordering criteria for the more frequently used medical X-ray procedures.
- Work with and through scientific, professional, and consumer organizations to promote discussion of consumer protection topics.
- Develop performance standards and conduct compliance programs for noncoherent light products.
- Accelerate the bioeffect research and development of measurement instrumentation in the ultrasound area.

State Agencies
- Strengthen the capability of the States in the regulation of consumer products.

J. Genetic Factors

1. The Problem

Approximately 4 percent of the live births in the United States annually have medical problems resulting from a genetic or partly genetic condition. These fall into three categories: chromosomal, Mendelian, and multifactorial. Studies have shown that genetic diseases account for a substantial proportion (20–29 percent) of the hospitalization in pediatric and adult populations. In 1971, 210,000 mentally retarded were housed in public institutions. Between 20 and 25 percent of these cases were attributable at least partly to genetic causes.

Chromosomal anomalies are associated with mental retardation, developmental abnormalities, multiple congenital malformations, and reduced survival. Approximately 1 of 200 newborns have chromosomal defects. The most common of the chromosomal defects is Down's syndrome, which affects approximately 1 in 600 births.

Mendelian disorders result in a diversity of abnormalities which in some cases are very mild and affect a single organ and, in other cases result in severe derangements and perinatal death. Some examples include cystic fibrosis which affects 1 in 4,000 Whites; sickle cell disease which affects 1 in 500 Blacks; and Tay Sachs disease which occurs in 1 of 3,600 live births among Ashkenazi Jews. Phenylketonuria (PKU) affects 1 in 15,000 live births. Screening at birth for PKU and galactosemia and appropriate diet therapy for those afflicted has virtually eliminated these conditions as causes of mental retardation.

Multifactorial disorders are attributed to the interaction of two or more genetic factors which individually may not be dangerous. Some disorders, such as anencephaly, are incompatible with life; others, such as cleft lip and palate and club foot, can usually be corrected. These affect between 1 to 10 per 1,000 births.

There are also genetic components in heart disease, hypertension, diabetes and schizophrenia.

2. Options

Legislation/Regulation/Enforcement

- Develop model State legislation for genetic screening. Such laws must ensure that the screening is medically appropriate, that the legal and civil rights of individuals are not infringed upon, and that ethical standards are maintained.
- Establish State Commissions or similar organizations to review and approve all new screening methods and to set standards to assure the quality of personnel and laboratories.
- In order to establish guidelines, undertake a PHS study of the ethical, legal, and social aspects of genetic diseases.

Research

- Support research to increase the number of diseases that can be diagnosed prenatally.

Maintenance

- Increase efforts to make prenatal diagnosis services available and to provide a system of quality assurance in laboratories performing such services.

Health Education

- Support education programs to alert the public to the possible risks of genetic diseases and to make them aware of the availability of counseling services to aid in dealing with these diseases.

K. Social-Psychological Factors

1. The Problem

An individual's health status is affected not only by the physical and biological environments, but also by his social environment. Causal relationships have not been demonstrated, but there are well established associations between rising unemployment or generally poor economic conditions, and increases in child abuse, crime, and, among some groups, increases in suicides and homicides.

These factors influence not only the person's psychological equilibrium but possibly his ability to resist disease as well. One theory suggests that disturbances within a person's cultural and social setting generates psychological stress, upsets the normal hormonal patterns of the individual, and thereby makes him more susceptible to disease.

The inability to deal with individual life crises (e.g., marriage, choice of job, difficult job situation, birth of a child) can lead to emotional disturbance, maladjustment, and mental illness. Although fully reliable figures do not exist, overall estimates indicate that no less than 10 percent of the U.S. population or 20 million people suffered from some form of mental illness in 1971.

One of the most striking social relationships is that of poverty (and low educational levels) and health status. Death rates, infant mortality rates, and morbidity rates are higher for the lower economic groups.

Racial groups also differ in incidences of various health problems although this is partly explained by the income differentials. The maternal mortality rate for non-white women in 1975 was 3.2 times higher than that of white women. The infant mortality rate in 1973 for whites was 15.8 compared with 26.5 per 100 live births for non-whites.

For young black males, homicide is the leading cause of death and continues to be a significant cause of death until middle age. In 1973 the homicide rate per 100,000 for non-white males was 65.8 compared with 8.3 for white males. Suicide rates, by contrast, are higher for whites. In 1973 they were 18.8 and 7.0 per 100,000 for white males and females, respectively, compared with rates of 10.0 for black males and 3.0 for black females.

Changes in the cultural values also seem to affect health. A number of theories have been advanced to explain changes in sexual attitudes, the drug culture, and the violence of the nineteen sixties—the war, decline in religious belief, affluence. While the causal links are uncertain, these forces have probably contributed to the greater incidence in venereal disease, deaths from violence among the young (suicides, homicides, motor vehicle accidents) and drug abuse.

It is virtually impossible to determine the prevalence for all abused drugs. A study in 1967 calculated opiate use at 108,424. Current (1974–1975) rates indicate that there are roughly between 600,000 and 800,000 narcotics users nationwide. According to NIDA, 74 percent of the drug users are between 10 and 29 years old and the two principal drugs used are marijuana and heroin. In 1973, there were an estimated 3,686 drug related deaths, one-third of these in the 20–29 year old group. Barbiturates and heroin/morphine accounted for approximately two-thirds of all these deaths in 1973.

The implications of these relationships between the social environment and health are far-reaching and argue for a preventive strategy which looks at fundamental problems in society—poverty side-by-side with affluence, changing values about drugs, sex, and violence, increased impersonality of society, and urbanization.

2. Options

Health Maintenance

- Develop mental health programs that give special emphasis and support to programs helping individuals to cope with life crises. Such programs would include anticipatory guidance, parent and family life education, health education, and counseling.
- Increase communications between mental health programs and family planning services, neighborhood health centers, schools and similar institutions to increase the potential for mental health promotion in these facilities.
- Support extensive research and demonstrations on techniques to prevent developmental failures in children, e.g., stimulating forms of preschool care, education of parents as enhancers of development, and intensive enrichment programs in early childhood.

Research

- Direct further research at understanding the mental health effects of urban processes on residents.
- Undertake research to devise practical chemical tests to detect individuals at risk of schizophrenia or the affective disorders before symptoms become manifest.

Modifying the Environment

- Undertake environmental sanitation measures focusing on problems of rats, lead-based paints, and dangerous conditions that lead to accidents.

II. ROLES IN PREVENTION

The broad view of prevention reflected in this theme, with its emphasis on primary prevention, necessarily goes beyond the boundaries of the health care system. It calls for the active involvement of the individual in reordering his way of living to a more healthful existence and it requires changes in how social and economic institutions use and interact with the environment. It also extends beyond the limits of the Department of Health, Education, and Welfare and of the Federal Government.

A. Federal

The Federal role in prevention is based on the assumption that most health problems can be more often effectively dealt with locally. The Public Health Service responsibility, therefore, is to:

- Identify and call public attention to the major causes of disease and death in the country and recommend alternative ways to prevent or control them.
- Assist States and localities and the private sector to improve their capacities to deal with these problems.
- Provide short-term technical and specialized assistance and training in prevention techniques and procedures.
- Promulgate uniform national prevention objectives, standards, and norms for planning programs and assessing progress.
- Provide funds to States and localities to carry out their prevention programs;
- Assure that all people have equal access to preventive programs and that the programs preserve each person's rights and freedom of choice.
- Compile and publish data on the nature, extent, and consequences of the principal causes of death and disease.
- Conduct and support research on the etiology of preventable diseases and on techniques for the prevention or control of the principal causes of such diseases.

The Public Health Service role also includes working with other agencies of DHEW and elsewhere in the Federal Government to assure consistency in Federal policies and full recognition of the health effects of such policies. Particular attention will be given to maintaining close communications with the Environmental Protection Agency and the Departments of Agriculture and Transportation on such matters as toxic substances, environmental pollution, nutrition, and motor vehicle accidents.

B. State and Local Health Agencies

Success in primary prevention depends upon the active collaboration of all those sectors of the society that are concerned with or affect the health of people. Within the health field itself, much of what is now undertaken by the Public Health Service in prevention depends on the active participation or conduct of programs by State and local health agencies. These agencies conduct immunization programs, venereal disease case-finding, food inspections, rodent control, diagnostic laboratories and community health education. They regulate health facilities, youth camps and migrant labor facilities, and provide nutrition counseling, family planning, and maternal and child health services.

It is the policy of the Public Health Service to help these agencies improve their capacity to conduct prevention programs. As a prime resource for prevention activities, they should be closely involved in the planning of prevention programs and given Federal assistance, particularly for prevention programs relating to the environment, community health education, and disease control.

C. Private Sector

The private sector, including voluntary associations, hospitals, universities and the media, also has a major role to play in a prevention strategy. Its involvement will be crucial in generating community and National backing for prevention measures, and in heightening people's awareness of conditions in their economic and social environment, as well as in their personal life style, that can adversely affect their health.

Appendix W

National Consumer Health Information and Health Promotion Act of 1976 P.L. 94-317, Title I

Public Law 94-317
94th Congress, S. 1466
June 23, 1976

An Act

To amend the Public Health Service Act to provide authority for health information and health promotion programs, to revise and extend the authority for disease prevention and control programs, and to revise and extend the authority for venereal disease programs, and to amend the Lead-Based Paint Poisoning Prevention Act to revise and extend that Act.

Be it enacted by the Senate and House of Representatives of the United States of America in Congress assembled,

Public Health Service Act, amendments; Lead-Based Paint Poisoning Act, extension. National Consumer Health Information and Health Promotion Act of 1976. 42 USC 201 note.

TITLE I—HEALTH INFORMATION AND HEALTH PROMOTION

SHORT TITLE

SEC. 101. This title may be cited as the "National Consumer Health Information and Health Promotion Act of 1976".

AMENDMENT TO PUBLIC HEALTH SERVICE ACT

SEC. 102. The Public Health Service Act is amended by adding at the end thereof the following new title:

"TITLE XVII—HEALTH INFORMATION AND HEALTH PROMOTION

"GENERAL AUTHORITY

"SEC. 1701. (a) The Secretary shall—

"(1) formulate national goals, and a strategy to achieve such goals, with respect to health information and health promotion, preventive health services, and education in the appropriate use of health care;

"(2) analyze the necessary and available resources for implementing the goals and strategy formulated pursuant to paragraph (1), and recommend appropriate educational and quality assurance policies for the needed manpower resources identified by such analysis;

"(3) undertake and support necessary activities and programs to—

"(A) incorporate appropriate health education components into our society, especially into all aspects of education and health care,

"(B) increase the application and use of health knowledge, skills, and practices by the general population in its patterns of daily living, and

"(C) establish systematic processes for the exploration, development, demonstration, and evaluation of innovative health promotion concepts;

"(4) undertake and support research and demonstrations respecting health information and health promotion, preventive health services, and education in the appropriate use of health care;

42 USC 300u.

90 STAT. 695

73-541 (137) O

251

Pub. Law 94-317   June 23, 1976

"(5) undertake and support appropriate training in, and undertake and support appropriate training in the operation of programs concerned with, health information and health promotion, preventive health services, and education in the appropriate use of health care;

"(6) undertake and support, through improved planning and implementation of tested models and evaluation of results, effective and efficient programs respecting health information and health promotion, preventive health services, and education in the appropriate use of health care;

"(7) foster the exchange of information respecting, and foster cooperation in the conduct of, research, demonstration, and training programs respecting health information and health promotion, preventive health services, and education in the appropriate use of health care;

"(8) provide technical assistance in the programs referred to in paragraph (7); and

"(9) use such other authorities for programs respecting health information and health promotion, preventive health services, and education in the appropriate use of health care as are available and coordinate such use with programs conducted under this title.

Administration.
42 USC 300k-2.
The Secretary shall administer this title in a manner consistent with the national health priorities set forth in section 1502 and with health planning and resource development activities undertaken under titles XV and XVI.

42 USC 300k-1,
300o.
Appropriation
authorization.
"(b) For payments under grants and contracts under this title there are authorized to be appropriated $7,000,000 for the fiscal year ending September 30, 1977, $10,000,000 for the fiscal year ending September 30, 1978, and $14,000,000 for the fiscal year ending September 30, 1979.

Grant or contract.
"(c) No grant may be made or contract entered into under this title unless an application therefor has been submitted to and approved by the Secretary. Such an application shall be submitted in such form and manner and contain such information as the Secretary may prescribe. Contracts may be entered into under this title without regard to sections 3648 and 3709 of the Revised Statutes (31 U.S.C. 529; 41 U.S.C. 5).

"RESEARCH PROGRAMS

42 USC 300u-1.
"SEC. 1702. (a) The Secretary is authorized to conduct and support by grant or contract (and encourage others to support) research in health information and health promotion, preventive health services, and education in the appropriate use of health care. Applications for grants and contracts under this section shall be subject to appropriate peer review. The Secretary shall also—

"(1) provide consultation and technical assistance to persons who need help in preparing research proposals or in actually conducting research;

"(2) determine the best methods of disseminating information concerning personal health behavior, preventive health services and the appropriate use of health care and of affecting behavior so that such information is applied to maintain and improve health, and prevent disease, reduce its risk, or modify its course or severity;

"(3) determine and study environmental, occupational, social, and behavioral factors which affect and determine health and ascertain those programs and areas for which educational and preventive measures could be implemented to improve health as it is affected by such factors;

June 23, 1976   Pub. Law 94-317

"(4) develop (A) methods by which the cost and effectiveness of activities respecting health information and health promotion, preventive health services, and education in the appropriate use of health care, can be measured, including methods for evaluating the effectiveness of various settings for such activities and the various types of persons engaged in such activities, (B) methods for reimbursement or payment for such activities, and (C) models and standards for the conduct of such activities, including models and standards for the education, by providers of institutional health services, of individuals receiving such services respecting the nature of the institutional health services provided the individuals and the symptoms, signs, or diagnoses which led to provision of such services;

"(5) develop a method for assessing the cost and effectiveness of specific medical services and procedures under various conditions of use, including the assessment of the sensitivity and specificity of screening and diagnostic procedures; and

"(6) enumerate and assess, using methods developed under paragraph (5), preventive health measures and services with respect to their cost and effectiveness under various conditions of use.

"(b) The Secretary shall make a periodic survey of the needs,   Survey.
interest, attitudes, knowledge, and behavior of the American public regarding health and health care. The Secretary shall take into consideration the findings of such surveys and the findings of similar surveys conducted by national and community health education organizations, and other organizations and agencies for formulating policy respecting health information and health promotion, preventive health services, and education in the appropriate use of health care.

"COMMUNITY PROGRAMS

"SEC. 1703. (a) The Secretary is authorized to conduct and support   42 USC 300u-2.
by grant or contract (and encourage others to support) new and innovative programs in health information and health promotion, preventive health services, and education in the appropriate use of health care, and may specifically—

"(1) support demonstration and training programs in such matters which programs (A) are in hospitals, ambulatory care settings, home care settings, schools, day care programs for children, and other appropriate settings representative of broad cross sections of the population, and include public education activities of voluntary health agencies, professional medical societies, and other private nonprofit health organizations, (B) focus on objectives that are measurable, and (C) emphasize the prevention or moderation of illness or accidents that appear controllable through individual knowledge and behavior;

"(2) provide consultation and technical assistance to organizations that request help in planning, operating, or evaluating programs in such matters;

"(3) develop health information and health promotion materials and teaching programs including (A) model curriculums for the training of educational and health professionals and paraprofessionals in health education by medical, dental, and nursing schools, schools of public health, and other institutions engaged in training of educational or health professionals, (B) model curriculums to be used in elementary and secondary schools and institutions of higher learning, (C) materials and programs

Pub. Law 94-317   June 23, 1976

for the continuing education of health professionals and paraprofessionals in the health education of their patients, (D) materials
for public service use by the printed and broadcast media, and
(E) materials and programs to assist providers of health care in
providing health education to their patients; and

"(4) support demonstration and evaluation programs for
individual and group self-help programs designed to assist the
participant in using his individual capacities to deal with health
problems, including programs concerned with obesity, hypertension, and diabetes.

Grants.

"(b) The Secretary is authorized to make grants to States and
other public and nonprofit private entities to assist them in meeting
the costs of demonstrating and evaluating programs which provide
information respecting the costs and quality of health care or information respecting health insurance policies and prepaid health plans,
or information respecting both. After the development of models pursuant to sections 1704(4) and 1704(5) for such information, no grant
may be made under this subsection for a program unless the information to be provided under the program is provided in accordance with
one of such models applicable to the information.

"(c) The Secretary is authorized to support by grant or contract
(and to encourage others to support) private nonprofit entities working in health information and health promotion, preventive health
services, and education in the appropriate use of health care. The
amount of any grant or contract for a fiscal year beginning after September 30, 1978, for an entity may not exceed 25 per centum of the
expenses of the entity for such fiscal year for health information and
health promotion, preventive health services, and education in the
appropriate use of health care.

"INFORMATION PROGRAMS

42 USC 300u-3.

"SEC. 1704. The Secretary is authorized to conduct and support by
grant or contract (and encourage others to support) such activities as
may be required to make information respecting health information
and health promotion, preventive health services, and education in
the appropriate use of health care available to the consumers of medical
care, providers of such care, schools, and others who are or should be
informed respecting such matters. Such activities may include at least
the following:

"(1) The publication of information, pamphlets, and other
reports which are specially suited to interest and instruct the
health consumer, which information, pamphlets, and other reports
shall be updated annually, shall pertain to the individual's ability to improve and safeguard his own health; shall include
material, accompanied by suitable illustrations, on child care,
family life and human development, disease prevention (particularly prevention of pulmonary disease, cardiovascular disease,
and cancer), physical fitness, dental health, environmental health,
nutrition, safety and accident prevention, drug abuse and alcoholism, mental health, management of chronic diseases (including
diabetes and arthritis), and venereal diseases; and shall be
designed to reach populations of different languages and of different social and economic backgrounds.

"(2) Securing the cooperation of the communications media,
providers of health care, schools, and others in activities designed
to promote and encourage the use of health maintaining information and behavior.

June 23, 1976   Pub. Law 94-317

"(3) The study of health information and promotion in advertising and the making to concerned Federal agencies and others such recommendations respecting such advertising as are appropriate.

"(4) The development of models and standards for the publication by States, insurance carriers, prepaid health plans, and others (except individual health practitioners) of information for use by the public respecting the cost and quality of health care, including information to enable the public to make comparisons of the cost and quality of health care.

"(5) The development of models and standards for the publication by States, insurance carriers, prepaid health plans, and others of information for use by the public respecting health insurance policies and prepaid health plans, including information on the benefits provided by the various types of such policies and plans, the premium charges for such policies and plans, exclusions from coverage or eligibility for coverage, cost sharing requirements, and the ratio of the amounts paid as benefits to the amounts received as premiums and information to enable the public to make relevant comparisons of the costs and benefits of such policies and plans.

"(6) Assess, with respect to the effectiveness, safety, cost, and required training for and conditions of use, of new aspects of health care, and new activities, programs, and services designed to improve human health and publish in readily understandable language for public and professional use such assessments and, in the case of controversial aspects of health care, activities, programs, or services, publish differing views or opinions respecting the effectiveness, safety, cost, and required training for and conditions of use, of such aspects of health care, activities, programs, or services.

"REPORT AND STUDY

"Sec. 1705. (a) The Secretary shall, not later than two years after the date of the enactment of this title and annually thereafter, submit to the President for transmittal to Congress a report on the status of health information and health promotion, preventive health services, and education in the appropriate use of health care. Each such report shall include—

42 USC 300u-4.

"(1) a statement of the activities carried out under this title since the last report and the extent to which each such activity achieves the purposes of this title;

"(2) an assessment of the manpower resources needed to carry out programs relating to health information and health promotion, preventive health services, and education in the appropriate use of health care, and a statement describing the activities currently being carried out under this title designed to prepare teachers and other manpower for such programs;

"(3) the goals and strategy formulated pursuant to section 1701(a)(1), the models and standards developed under this title, and the results of the study required by subsection (b) of this section; and

"(4) such recommendations as the Secretary considers appropriate for legislation respecting health information and health promotion, preventive health services, and education in the appropriate use of health care, including recommendations for revisions to and extension of this title.

Pub. Law 94-317   June 23, 1976

Study.

"(b) The Secretary shall conduct a study of health education services and preventive health services to determine the coverage of such services under public and private health insurance programs, including the extent and nature of such coverage and the cost sharing requirements required by such programs for coverage of such services.

"OFFICE OF HEALTH INFORMATION AND HEALTH PROMOTION"

Establishment.
42 USC 300u-5.

"SEC. 1706. The Secretary shall establish within the Office of the Assistant Secretary for Health an Office of Health Information and Health Promotion which shall—

"(1) coordinate all activities within the Department which relate to health information and health promotion, preventive health services, and education in the appropriate use of health care;

"(2) coordinate its activities with similar activities of organizations in the private sector; and

"(3) establish a national information clearinghouse to facilitate the exchange of information concerning matters relating to health information and health promotion, preventive health services, and education in the appropriate use of health care, to facilitate access to such information, and to assist in the analysis of issues and problems relating to such matters."

Index

A

257